101 TIPS FOR STAYING HEALTHY WITH DIABETES (& AVOIDING COMPLICATIONS)

▲

A project of
The American Diabetes Association

▼

Written and produced by
The University of New Mexico
Diabetes Care Team:

David S. Schade, M.D. *Editor in Chief*

Patrick J. Boyle, M.D.

Mark R. Burge, M.D.

Dena Robinson, R.N., C.D.E.

Virginia Valentine, R.N., M.S., C.D.E.

◣**. American Diabetes Association.**

Publisher
Susan H. Lau

Editorial Director
Peter Banks

Editor
Sherrye Landrum

Copyright © 1996 by American Diabetes Association.
All rights reserved.

Printed in the United States of America

AMERICAN DIABETES ASSOCIATION
1660 Duke Street
Alexandria, Virginia 22314

```
Library of Congress Cataloging-in-Publication Data

101 tips for staying healthy with diabetes (& avoiding complications)
  : a project of the American Diabetes Association / written and
produced by the University of New Mexico Diabetes Care Tam  :  David
S. Schade, editor-in-chief ... [et al.].
     p.    cm.
   ISBN 0-945448-71-6 (pbk.)
   1. Diabetes--Popular works.  2. Diabetes--Miscellannea.
I. Schade, David S., 1942-  .  II. University of New Mexico.
Diabetes Care Team.    III. American Diabetes association.
RC660.4.a16  1996
616.4'62--dc20                                    96-18928
          ISBN 0-945448-71-6                      CIP
```

**101 TIPS FOR STAYING HEALTHY WITH DIABETES
(& AVOIDING COMPLICATIONS)**

▼

TABLE OF CONTENTS

ACKNOWLEDGMENTS

▼

The University of New Mexico Diabetes Care Team wishes to acknowledge the editorial expertise of Carolyn King, M.Ed., of the University of New Mexico. We also acknowledge the editorial assistance of Ms. Sherrye Landrum of the American Diabetes Association and the graphic expertise of Wickham & Associates for the cover design of the book.

Thanks to Greg Edmondson for copyediting and to Francine Kaufman, MD, Eleanor Lordon, RN, MS, CNS, CDE, and David B. Kelley, MD, for reviewing the manuscript. A special thanks to Jim Stein at Insight Graphics for desktopping the manuscript and to Carolyn Segree for coordinating the printing.

CONTRIBUTORS

▼

The University of New Mexico Diabetes Care Team is composed of:

David S. Schade, M.D.	Diabetes Specialist
Patrick J. Boyle, M.D.	Diabetes Specialist
Mark R. Burge, M.D.	Diabetes Specialist
Virginia Valentine, R.N., M.S., C.D.E	Clinical Nurse Specialist/Diabetes
Dena Robinson, R.N., C.D.E.	Diabetes Case Manager
and Carolyn Kling, M.Ed.	Graphic Designer

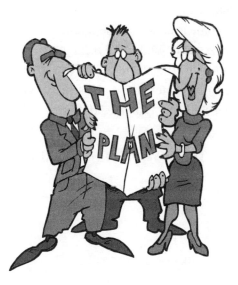

Introduction

▼

We were very pleased that our first book, *101 Tips for Improving Your Blood Sugar,* was so well received by people with diabetes. This first book was the result of suggestions made to us by our patients who had successfully found ways to reduce their blood sugars to appropriate target ranges. We then passed these suggestions to you, our readers. The current book, *101 Tips for Staying Healthy with Diabetes (& Avoiding Complications),* brings more of our patients' tips to you.

As health providers, we are convinced that the patient should make the important decisions concerning diabetes and health. To do this successfully, each person must understand both the reasons for the health goals and the ways to accomplish them. The format of our two books conveys our patients' tips through illustrations and text.

Diabetes treatment is undergoing rapid changes. Thanks to many dedicated individuals and organizations, additional options for treatment will continue to become available in the future. We are grateful to the American Diabetes Association for publishing our books and making them available to its members at a reduced cost. All proceeds from our books go to furthering diabetes care and research. With your help, we believe that diabetes will be a "curable" disease within the next 10 years. Thank you.

— The University of New Mexico Diabetes Care Team

Chapter One:
GENERAL INFORMATION

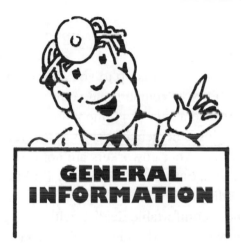

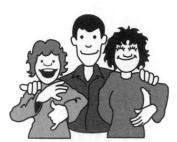

Should I tell my boss and coworkers that I have diabetes?

▼
TIP:

Whether or not to tell is up to you. You do have a responsibility to yourself and your coworkers to keep the work environment safe. It is important to have a system in place for managing emergencies, such as a severe low blood sugar or a sick day. Your coworkers are not responsible for taking care of you, but you will probably find that they will be very understanding and want to help you stay healthy. Most people feel more comfortable dealing with emergencies if they have some preparation and understanding. You don't have to make diabetes the daily topic of conversation, and you may feel uncomfortable letting people at work become the "control patrol." This is a personal choice that requires consideration on your part, but you will find that your life is easier if you allow others to support you in managing your diabetes and staying healthy.

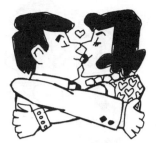

Can I catch diabetes from someone else?

▼
TIP:

No, you cannot. Diabetes is not like a cold or the flu. There are many causes of diabetes, but both types I & II have never been shown to be infectious or contagious (catchable). You cannot catch diabetes from another person, even by kissing them. Most diabetes develops from an inherited tendency to get it. If you have inherited this gene, you may develop type I diabetes when you are exposed to something in the environment. This unknown factor triggers the onset of diabetes. You may develop type II diabetes if (in addition to the gene) you gain weight and don't exercise regularly. There are also less common causes of diabetes, such as prolonged, excessive drinking of alcohol or having too much iron in your blood. Thus, there are many causes of diabetes, but catching it from another person is not one of them.

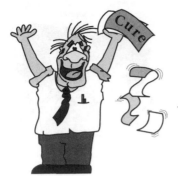

*H*ow close are we to a cure for
diabetes?

▼
TIP:

It depends on what you mean by "cure." Diabetes is not really one disease. It probably has many causes and therefore
many cures. Much progress has been made in the last few
years toward prevention of diabetes and treatment of the disease once it occurs. These advances are important until a cure
is available. The ultimate cure for diabetes would probably be
a replacement of the cells of the pancreas that make insulin.
This could be done by inserting a remote-controlled insulin
pump that is automatically regulated by a glucose sensor. The
implantable pump has already been developed and tested in
more than 400 people worldwide. Glucose sensors are under
development and should be available within the next several
years.

Another approach is to transplant insulin-producing cells
into the person with diabetes. This approach has already been
done successfully in animals with diabetes. It has been more
difficult in humans because humans tend to kill off these cells,
because our body sees them as foreign material. Many
researchers are trying to overcome these problems. What we
can say is that we expect a cure for some types of diabetes
within the next ten years.

D *oes diabetes put me at risk for developing thyroid problems?*

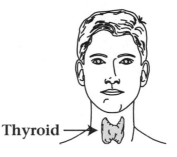

Thyroid

▼
TIP:

Perhaps. The thyroid gland in your neck secretes thyroid hormone. Low levels of thyroid hormone (thyroid failure) are common in individuals with insulin dependent diabetes (type I). Thyroid hormone gives you energy and helps maintain other organ systems in your body. We recommend that you get a blood test for thyroid hormone once a year, particularly if you feel more tired than usual or have other symptoms such as constipation, dry skin, and feeling cold most of the time. Treatment is easy and inexpensive. This is important, because low thyroid hormone that goes untreated can lead to many medical problems. Do not hesitate to ask your doctor periodically to check your blood thyroid hormone level. Remember that other medical problems can occur in people with diabetes that are not directly related to high blood sugar levels.

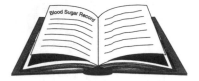

*H*ow can I make the most
of my visit with my
health-care team?

▼
TIP:

irst, plan ahead. Write down on paper all the questions that
you want to ask the team. It is too easy to forget your questions if you don't write them down. Also bring along a pencil
or pen to write down the answers. If you're prepared, the visit
is more likely to meet your needs. Second, show up for your
appointment on time. If you are late, your health-care team may
not be able to spend enough time with you to solve your problems. (For waiting room reading, you could bring this book or
our first book, *101 Tips for Improving Your Blood Sugar*, and
review the tips that apply to you.) Third, always bring in all
your current medications so that the health-care team can check
them. This will ensure that you don't run out of medication and
that the pharmacy gives you the medication that your doctor
prescribes. Fourth, be sure and bring in records of your recent
blood sugars, weight, blood pressure, and exercise schedule.
These records help you and the team see your progress in meet-
ing your goals. If you don't have a logbook, bring your blood
sugar meter.

*H*ow often should I plan on seeing my doctor to be as healthy as I can be?

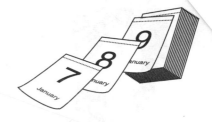

▼
TIP:

The frequency of medical visits required for your diabetes will vary according to how long you've had diabetes, your ability to effectively adjust your treatment regimen to maintain good blood sugar control, and whether you have diabetic complications or other medical problems which may interfere with your diabetes management.

At a minimum, all diabetic patients should plan on seeing a doctor twice a year. Recharging your motivation to achieve good blood sugar control is an important part of every visit. You should have an HbA_{1c} test done then, or if you are on insulin, you should have the test done quarterly to see how your blood glucose control is doing.

Plus, every patient with diabetes should have someone they can contact on short notice to discuss problems as they arise, such as unexplained high blood sugars or sudden illness. This person need not be a physician, but may be a certified diabetes educator, nurse practitioner, or nurse case manager.

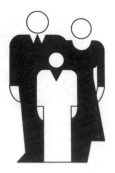

S *hould members of my family read this book?*

▼
TIP:

Yes! There are several good reasons for each member of your family to read this book. First, there are many tips that apply equally well to people with or without diabetes. Anyone who wants to stay in good health will benefit from these tips. Second, your family members can support you better when they understand what is needed. For example, a change to eating healthier meals is easier if all family members make the same commitment. There are outdated ideas of what is good for a person with diabetes. Keeping up-to-date makes it easier to plan family outings, picnics, and parties with you in mind. Each family member should be able to recognize the signs and symptoms of low blood sugar. Third, family members of people with diabetes have a higher risk of developing diabetes themselves. By changing to a healthier lifestyle, you and your family members, we believe, will prevent or significantly delay the onset of diabetes.

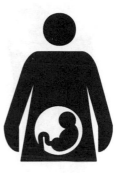

*D*oes getting diabetes when I am *pregnant mean that I am more likely to get permanent diabetes later?*

▼

TIP:

Yes. The fact that you get high blood sugars during pregnancy indicates that your pancreas cannot make enough extra insulin to cover the increased needs caused by pregnancy. This suggests that you might develop diabetes even if you never get pregnant again. Approximately 5% of women like you will develop diabetes each year if they don't make efforts to improve their lifestyles. Women gain weight during pregnancy but do not always lose all of it after delivery. With several pregnancies, a woman may gain quite a bit of weight. Therefore, if you develop high blood sugars during pregnancy, it is most important that you lose all of the weight you gained during your pregnancy. Eat healthy meals and exercise daily. This is the best approach you can take to prevent permanent diabetes from occurring.

If you decide to breastfeed, do not begin a weight loss program without medical advice. To breastfeed you need the same amount of calories that you needed during the last 3 months of your pregnancy. When you have stopped breastfeeding, focus on losing any extra weight that you still have.

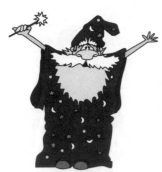

*I*s *diabetes a new disease?*

▼
TIP:

No. Diabetes was known two thousand years ago when Aretaeus of Cappadocia, the Greek physician, named it. However, very little progress was made in understanding or treating the disease until 1869 when Paul Langerhans described small islands (islets) in the pancreas. However, he did not know their function. Things progressed more rapidly when Oskar Minkowski realized that removing the pancreas from a dog caused the dog to urinate frequently. He also found sugar in the dog's urine. In 1909, the Belgian scientist Jean de Meyer used the term "insulin" for a hypothetical substance in the pancreas which controls blood sugar even though insulin had not yet been discovered. Finally in 1921, after a series of experiments, J.J.R. Macleod, Charles Best, Frederick Banting, and James Collip succeeded in purifying insulin and successfully treating a diabetic patient with it. This discovery, after two thousand years, saved many people from dying in a coma due to high blood sugars. Diabetes has been around a long time, but we still need new and better therapies.

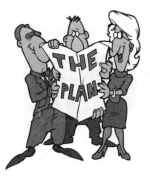

*W*hat is my "health-care team" and how can I find these health providers?

▼
TIP:

In addition to your doctor, you need someone trained to help you with the day-to-day challenges of living with diabetes. Diabetes educator nurses and dietitians, plus your doctor, are the core members of your health-care team. A Certified Diabetes Educator (CDE) is a health professional (registered nurse (RN), registered dietitian (RD), pharmacist, physician, etc.) who has been trained and "certified" as an expert in diabetes education and management. If you cannot find a CDE, you may find a nurse or dietitian interested in diabetes and willing to help you. Ask your doctor if he or she knows someone with diabetes experience. You can get a list of CDEs in your area by calling the American Association of Diabetes Educators at (800) 338-3633. You may also want to look for a diabetes education program that offers individual or group classes. Your local American Diabetes Association chapter has a list of "recognized" diabetes centers in your area. The phone number is in the white pages of the phone book. If there isn't a recognized diabetes center near you, call your local hospital and ask about a diabetes education program or diabetes educators on staff.

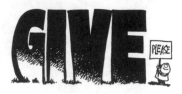 *What can I do to help cure diabetes?*

▼
TIP:

You can do a lot! Most people don't realize how important their effort can be in helping to cure diabetes. The main reason that so much progress has been made in the last 50 years is the work of individuals like you supporting organizations searching for the cure for diabetes. These organizations include the American Diabetes Association and the Juvenile Diabetes Foundation International.

At the local level, you can encourage friends and neighbors to support fund-raising efforts by your local diabetes chapters, such as walking events. Donations to these organizations will support new research in diabetes and are deductible from your income tax. Joining one of these organizations will connect you to up-to-date information on better diabetes management. They will also keep you informed of important legislation concerning diabetes in the U.S. Congress. Your letters to your local and state representatives (Congressmen and Senators) can definitely help make state and national monies available for diabetes research and treatment. Your local American Diabetes Association Affiliate can provide you with their names and addresses. Remember, you really can make a difference.

*I*s diabetes a dangerous disease?

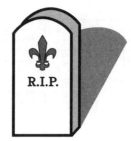

▼
TIP:

Yes, it is. There are statistics to prove that diabetes causes much suffering and loss of time from work. For example, it is the leading cause of kidney failure in this country. In addition, 15,000 to 30,000 people each year lose their eyesight because of diabetes. This year 160,000 individuals will die from diabetes-related causes in the United States. In fact, according to experts, during the last 20 years, diabetes has caused more deaths than all of the wars throughout the world in the last century. Unfortunately, the situation is getting worse, not better, because of the increasing number of people with diabetes. We all need to do our best to prevent and to treat this disease in the U.S. and throughout the world.

The results of the Diabetes Control and Complications Trial (DCCT) show that we can live healthier lives with diabetes by keeping blood glucose levels near normal. Modern advances in self testing and treatment make this possible.

		D	E	M	E	T	R	I	U	S
		I								
S	U	G	A	R		U				
		B				R				
	M	E	L	L	I	T	U	S		
		T				N		W		
W	A	T	E	R		E		E		
		S						L		
								L		

What does the name diabetes mellitus mean?

▼
TIP:

The names diabetes and mellitus come from two different places. The first name, diabetes, is usually attributed to the Greek physician Aretaeus, who lived in 200 BC. He used the term diabetes, meaning siphon or to flow through, for a disease in which the water that a person drinks runs rapidly through his/her body. His patients sucked in water at one end and emptied it at the other. It was not until the end of the 18th century that the term mellitus was added to diabetes. An Englishman, John Rollo, and a German, Johann Peter Frank, first used the term mellitus (which means sweet as honey) in the medical literature to describe the sweet taste of the urine. So to answer your question, the name diabetes mellitus means a medical condition in which the patient drinks too much water and urinates frequently. The urine is sweet because it contains sugar.

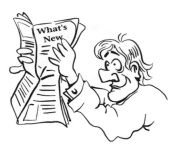

*H*ow can I know if a new diabetes product is right for me?

▼
TIP:

This is one time when being a skeptic is a good idea. Many times, news releases make a product sound like it will work for everyone, but in fact it may be useful for specific conditions only. In the United States we have many regulations to protect us from unproved (and possibly dangerous) new treatments. The Food and Drug Administration has strict guidelines regarding the research and testing that must be done on a new drug or therapy before it can be sold to the public. Many times you will read reports about a new product or drug while it is still in the early phases of testing. Testing takes several years. If safety problems or side effects are found during the testing, the product will not be marketed. Your health-care team may have information on new products, so you should check with them when something new is available. They will help you make a decision as to whether the new product is right for you.

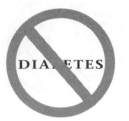

*C*an diabetes be prevented?

▼
TIP:

Many scientists believe that the answer is "yes." Because the causes of type I and type II diabetes are different, approaches to preventing each form of diabetes are different.

Type I diabetes is thought to be caused by an allergic-like reaction, probably to insulin, the pancreas, and/or some substance in the pancreas. If this is true, then it is possible that diabetes could be prevented by giving the susceptible person small injections of insulin, much like allergy shots may prevent hay fever. This approach has been successful in animals who were bred to get diabetes. The National Institute of Health (NIH) is currently conducting a nationwide study to test this promising possibility.

Type II diabetes does not seem to be caused by an allergic reaction. The cause is probably related to a hereditary defect which reduces a person's sensitivity to insulin. New medications used early may prevent type II diabetes. Also lifestyle changes (exercise and weight loss) may reverse this defect and prevent it. The U.S. government is testing this promising approach in another nationwide study. Within the next 5 to 10 years, we should know the answer to your question.

*I*s there a time of year when my
family or I am more likely to get
diabetes?

AUTUMN

▼
TIP:

Yes and no. Many studies have been done to determine when people get diabetes.

Type I diabetes (often called insulin dependent diabetes) usually occurs in thin individuals less than 30 years of age. It is more common to develop type I diabetes in the fall of the year, which happens to be the season in which many viral infections occur (for example, chicken pox, flu, and measles). The higher rate of type I diabetes during the fall months has been used to suggest that type I diabetes may be started by a virus that causes an infection. Whether this is true or not has not been found.

Type II diabetes (often called non insulin dependent diabetes) usually occurs in overweight people over the age of 30 years. There does not seem to be a seasonal increase in the development of type II diabetes. This difference in the time of year that diabetes develops is one of the many ways the two types of diabetes are not alike.

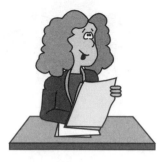

Why do I have a pre-existing condition rider attached to my health insurance policy that excludes any coverage for my diabetes for one year?

▼
TIP:

Insurance companies separate people into groups depending on their "risk" (the chance that they will cost money to the insurance company). Because diabetes is expensive to manage and because diabetes is associated with other serious diseases, insurance companies feel that they should either charge you more or not cover you for the first year. In this first year with pre-existing conditions excluded, you must try to find a way to protect yourself from excessive health-care expenses. Before you change jobs, be sure to consider the complete health benefit package of both jobs. Consider the impact your new job may have on your present health benefits package. You may be able to retain insurance coverage from your previous position by selecting your COBRA benefit, which is required by law to allow you to continue your insurance for 18 months. You should also check with your State Insurance Commission to find out if your state has an insurance program for people who are uninsurable because they have a chronic disease. If you are unable to afford insurance or health-care costs, many county/state supported hospitals have funds that are available to help with medical costs.

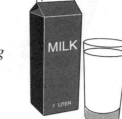

*I*s it true that drinking cow's milk during
infancy causes diabetes?

▼
TIP:

We don't know. The protein in milk may be one of the environmental triggers for diabetes. A group of researchers in Canada and Finland found that children who are diagnosed with type I diabetes were more likely to have been fed cow's milk during their first 6 months of life than a group of children who did not develop diabetes. Their immune systems attacked a protein found in the milk. This protein "looks" like beta cells—those cells that make insulin. It may be that the body's immune system mistakenly identifies its own beta cells as the milk protein and attacks them, too. Although these results are interesting, other research has not found that drinking cow's milk during the first year of life is a cause of diabetes. Further research must be done before we find an answer to this question.

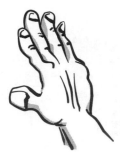

Why are my fingernails thick and pulling away from the nail bed?

▼
TIP:

You may have a fungal infection of your fingernails. Fungal infections of the skin, such as "athlete's foot," are more common in people with diabetes. These fungal infections can occasionally involve unusual areas of the body, such as your nails, scalp, or groin. A fungal infection of your fingernails is not a serious threat to your overall health, but it may make your nails brittle and unsightly. You can also spread the infection to other areas of your body, such as your scalp, by scratching with infected nails.

You should see your health-care team or a dermatologist to have your infection treated. They can take a sample from under your nails and examine it under the microscope to confirm the diagnosis. Nail infections are difficult to cure, however, and you will probably require treatment with an oral drug for several months. Because these drugs may damage your liver or bone marrow, you may need to have blood tests every few weeks to monitor your blood cell counts and your liver function. After all of this effort, you may be rewarded with a return of healthy fingernails.

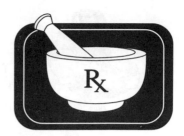

A *re there any new treatments for*
type II diabetes?

▼
TIP:

Yes, there are two new therapies which may help people with diabetes who do not need to take insulin. Both of these treatments were approved for use by the Food and Drug Administration in 1995. These medications are exciting advances because they work in ways different from presently available treatments. These new medications can be combined with older treatments to make control of blood sugar easier. The good news about these medications is that they do not cause weight gain even when their use improves glucose control.

The first new medication is metformin (Glucophage®), a drug used in Europe for many years. It is usually taken twice a day. The second medication, acarbose (Precose®), is usually taken before each meal. It slows the absorption of carbohydrate from your intestine, which makes it easier for your own insulin to control the rise in blood sugar after a meal. (This medicine is sometimes called a "starch blocker.") The main side effect of each of these medications is stomach upset and sometimes bloating or diarrhea. Discuss these medications with your health-care team to see if they will help you meet your blood sugar goals.

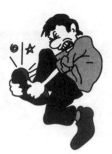

*S*hould I be concerned about a small
*red blister on my foot from walking
in new shoes?*

▼
TIP:

Yes! You may look at a small blister and think that it is
nothing serious, but it can be. If it breaks, this blister in
the skin can allow germs into your foot. These germs can
cause not only an infection in your foot, but also in the bone.
Infections in the bone are very difficult to treat and often are
the cause of amputations. What you should do right now is to
carefully wash your feet in gentle soap and water and dry thor-
oughly. Then put a small amount of antibiotic ointment on a
dressing and cover the wound. Next, call your health-care team
and let them know that you have a sore on your foot. Your
health-care team will want to see your foot to decide if you
need to get started on an antibiotic medication. Finally, quit
wearing the shoes that caused the blister. Purchase of a comfortable pair of shoes is one of the best investments you can
make. The shoes you wear must fit your feet. Careful attention
now can prevent future problems.

A m I more likely to develop skin infections because I have diabetes?

▼
TIP:

Y ou may be. People with diabetes who are overweight or who have high blood sugars most of the time are more likely to develop skin infections than thin people with normal blood sugars. High blood sugars can interfere with your body's natural defense systems. Once they start, some of these infections can spread rapidly, causing fever, chills, and tiredness. It is very important that you examine your skin each day and promptly take care of any ulcers, redness, or skin breakdowns which may be new. Yeast infections usually occur in warm, moist areas of the body, particularly in the genital region, under breasts, and between folds of skin. Infections of the face, foot, and ear canal may be particularly serious and should be checked by your health-care team. Many different types of treatment are available for these skin problems, and you should ask for advice before applying drugstore skin creams. Good skin care is essential for good health.

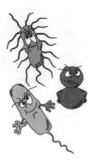

*C*an my diabetes cause diarrhea?

▼
TIP:

Yes. Frequent diarrhea occurs in 5 to 20% of people with long-standing diabetes. The possible causes include fewer digestive enzymes being released from the pancreas, overuse of magnesium-containing antacids, or too many bacteria in the upper part of the intestine (where they should not normally be). Often, however, the cause is unknown. Damage to the nerves which control movement in the bowel is thought to be the cause. Have an evaluation by your health-care team. For example, if you don't have enough digestive enzymes, a pill taken with meals may cure the problem. If the cause of your diarrhea remains unknown, there are still treatments which may increase the hardness of your stools and decrease the number of daily bowel movements. Some of these treatments include simple over-the-counter remedies like psyllium (Metamucil®), or a kaolin and pectin mixture (Kaopectate®). Other people respond to prescription drugs, such as cholesterol-binding resins (cholestyramine), antibiotics (tetracycline or erythromycin), or drugs designed to decrease movement in the bowel like loperamide (Lomotil®). Whatever the cause of your diarrhea, you deserve a careful medical review of this problem, because chances are good that some of your symptoms can be relieved.

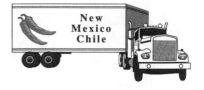

Could I lose my job driving a truck if I start insulin?

▼
TIP:

If you can prove that your diabetes is in good control with blood glucose records and glycated hemoglobin test (HbA$_{1c}$) results, you may be able to continue in the job in your state. Individual state governments have rules for jobs driving automobiles, trucks, or commercial vehicles within that state. Within an individual state, most jobs are reviewed on a case by case basis.

However, the U.S. Dept. of Transportation, Federal Highway Administration governs driving commercial vehicles between states. Their policy is that "A person is physically qualified to drive a motor vehicle if s/he has no established medical history or clinical diagnosis of diabetes mellitus currently requiring insulin for control." This would prevent you from driving a truck across state lines if you are taking insulin. You should contact your State Department of Transportation to see what your state's policy is on various occupations that rely on driving ability within that state.

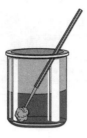

Should I test my urine for glucose and ketones?

▼
TIP:

Sometimes. It is not an accurate way to measure blood sugar. It is the way to check for ketones when you cannot eat or are ill. A buildup of ketones tells you that you are developing ketoacidosis. Ketones are breakdown products of fat which produce acid in the body. Too much acid can result in hospitalization. Therefore, when you are sick with a cold or the flu, you should test your urine for ketones and call your health-care team if you detect any. You can buy urine ketone testing strips at the drugstore.

The information about blood glucose that you get from urine testing of sugar is not precise enough to make decisions for treatment. Your kidney does not spill sugar into your urine until your blood sugar is higher than 200 mg/dl. The American Diabetes Association does not recommend you use urine sugar testing (especially if you're taking insulin) if you can perform finger stick blood testing.

*I*s there information on the Internet
about diabetes?

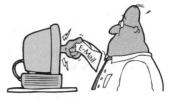

▼
TIP:

Yes, there is. You can keep yourself current on the latest
information about diabetes electronically by using either
your telephone or your computer. The Diabetes Information
and Action Line (D.I.A.L.) provides general information on
diabetes for anyone who calls. Last year, more than 250,000
people called the American Diabetes Association (ADA) for
information with a toll-free number: 1-800-DIABETES.
Another place for you to get information is on the Internet and
the World Wide Web. The ADA, with America Online,
launched an online diabetes forum in June 1995. America
Online subscribers can look at information on various topics,
including exercise, diabetes self-care, research, and ADA
activities. To get to this forum, type the keywords "American
Diabetes." The ADA also has a page on the World Wide Web.
If you use the Internet, you can call up the official ADA home
page at http://www.diabetes.org to obtain information on
ADA's activities, policies, and research programs.

Chapter Two:
GLUCOSE CONTROL

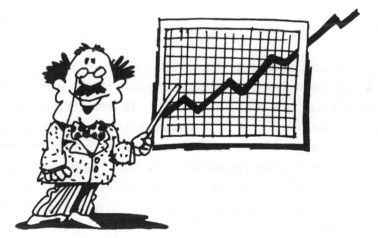

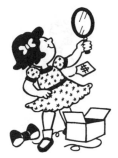

*W*hy can't I get my 8-year-old
daughter to help take care of her
diabetes?

▼
TIP:

Because it is difficult and frustrating for her to do it. Young
children usually are unable to assume full responsibility
for their diabetes care until they reach the teenage years. In
fact, an eight-year-old child cannot understand something as
complicated as a chronic disease, and she may actually blame
herself for the fact that she has diabetes. She may be more
timid than other children her age and worry more than usual
when you are apart from her ("separation anxiety").

She has new and challenging tasks every day, like going to
school and making new friends, so she may not be interested
in caring for her diabetes. She needs to feel secure in her daily
activities and let you care for her diabetes for now. It may help
her self-confidence if she succeeds at doing some of the basic
tasks such as blood glucose checks and keeping her log book.
Discuss with your health-care team how flexible her schedule
can be and the appropriate goals for her diabetes control. You
may find that you can loosen up on her control somewhat in
the interest of safety and convenience. Remember that the day
is coming when your daughter will be able to care for her
diabetes herself, and she'll only need your help occasionally.
Just don't rush her.

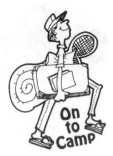

*H*ow can I help my 13-year-old son
cope with his diabetes?

▼
TIP:

Unfortunately, this is a hectic period for him and diabetes care may seem to be low on his priority list. The onset of puberty can complicate diabetes care. He may have a dramatic increase in insulin requirements over a short period of time. Turn over the responsibility for diabetes care to your son gradually as he is ready to accept it. You will both need to be flexible to adjust to all the demands on him.

It is possible that your son may be more open to learning from his peers than from you during the coming years. Help him get together with other teenagers who have diabetes so he can see the various ways they cope with diabetes. Diabetes summer camp provides an excellent opportunity for this. Your son will see both healthy and unhealthy behaviors at camp, but he'll be encouraged to manage his own diabetes with experience and knowledge. Every state has a diabetes summer camp with a full medical staff. The friendships that develop at camp are often strong and can last a lifetime. Contact your local chapter of the American Diabetes Association for more information about a camp in your area.

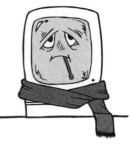

What can I take for a cold since it seems that all the cold medicines at the drugstore are labeled "not for people with diabetes"?

▼
TIP:

Probably the best thing to do about a cold is to take acetaminophen (Tylenol®) for the aches, pains, or fever, get plenty of rest, and drink lots of fluids. Be sure to check your blood sugar often and be ready to respond to a rise in your blood sugar. You and your health-care team need to set up a sick-day plan. Then you'll know better what to eat or drink, when to test your blood glucose and ketones, and when to call them for help.

Drugs that help reduce the symptoms of a cold are cough medicines, antihistamines (block allergic reaction), and decongestants (reduce swelling in the nose). The cough medicines and antihistamines tend to make you very sleepy. Chemicals in decongestants work in your swollen sinus tissues by making the blood vessels narrower and thus reducing blood flow. This may help your runny nose, but if you have heart disease or very poor circulation, they can cause serious problems. These medications may be perfectly OK for you if your heart is healthy and you have good circulation. However, if you have diabetes, the label warns you to talk to your doctor before taking this medicine.

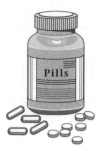

*W*ill the medication I am taking for
depression affect my blood sugar?

▼
TIP:

Probably not. Depression is more common in patients with
chronic diseases like diabetes—up to 40% of people with
diabetes may have depression at some point in their lives.
Medications for depression have no major direct impact on
how your oral diabetes medications or insulin work to control
your blood sugar.

On the other hand, keeping diabetes management at the top
of your list of things to deal with can seem impossible if you
are depressed. While there are many ways of dealing with
depression, sometimes several months of treatment with
medication can allow you to get back to being yourself faster.
A vicious cycle can develop where high blood sugars make
you feel sleepy and as though you don't have enough energy to
get out and exercise. The exercise would help bring the blood
glucose down. Dealing with depression can break the cycle
and put you back on track, eating right and exercising, to help
you feel better all the time.

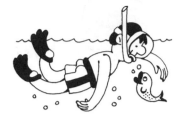

*B*ecause I have arthritis in my
hips, can you recommend
exercises other than walking?

▼
TIP:

Many people with arthritic pain in their hips or knees cannot take the 30- to 60-minute walk that is recommended to improve blood sugar control. You can do armchair aerobics and stretches while sitting. Water aerobics in the swimming pool is another activity that does not put stress on your joints. All exercise routines should include a 10-minute warm-up period, 10 to 30 minutes of exercise, and a 10-minute cool-down period. The exercise must be intense enough to get your heart rate up but not so intense that you can't speak. You may break out in a light sweat (if you're not in a pool).

Weight loss is not the only benefit of exercising. Exercise also increases insulin sensitivity, improves blood flow to the heart and muscles, and helps improve blood sugar control. As with all exercise programs, you should consult your health-care team for recommendations about the activity that is right for you. Don't let your arthritis prevent you from exercising.

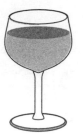

Is it acceptable for me to have a glass of wine with dinner?

▼
TIP:

It may be. Alcohol can cause severe, life-threatening low blood sugar, even in people who do not have diabetes. That is why we say drink only with food. There is evidence that small amounts of alcohol are OK for people with diabetes if you are not pregnant or do not have a history of alcohol abuse. For example, one recent study shows that moderate alcohol intake (no more than 1 drink a day) is associated with lower blood sugar levels and improved insulin sensitivity in healthy people who do not have diabetes. Another study shows that blood sugar levels do not differ for 12 hours after a *meal* between diabetic patients (both types I and II) who drink a shot of vodka before dinner, or a glass of wine with dinner, or a shot of cognac after dinner and those who drink an equal amount of water. Finally, a number of studies have suggested that moderate alcohol intake may have a positive effect on blood cholesterol and lipid levels. Just remember that alcohol calories should be included in your meal plan and have your one drink with food.

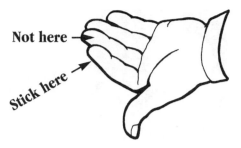

Not here →

Stick here →

How can I reduce the pain of frequent finger sticks?

▼
TIP:

One technique is to stick the side of your finger where there are fewer pain sensors instead of sticking directly into your fingerpad. Another technique is to use an automatic (spring loaded) lancet holder which can vary how deep the lancet goes. Use the shortest depth that will give you an adequate drop of blood for testing. Since skin thickness varies from person to person, you'll need to try different depths to see what works for you.

Because of the danger of transmitting hepatitis and other blood-borne diseases, never "borrow" another person's device. Hopefully, in the next few years, noninvasive blood sugar monitors will become available for you to use. These monitors will shine a light beam through the skin to read the amount of sugar in your blood. Because of the great need and demand for these monitors, it isn't a question of whether they will be available, but when. Keep in touch with your health-care team for information in this area.

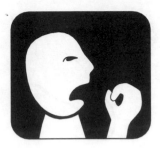

Why do I yawn when I have low blood sugar?

▼
TIP:

Probably because low blood sugar makes you feel tired. The classical signs and symptoms of low blood sugar include sweating, hunger, nervousness, and agitation. However, many people with diabetes do not have the usual symptoms. Some people have no symptoms at all! Other people have unusual symptoms of low blood sugar. In some people, a change in their personality can occur so that they become hostile and combative. Some people simply look "glassy-eyed," "spacey," or are mildly confused. It is very important to know what your low blood sugar symptoms are so that your friends and family will know when to help you.

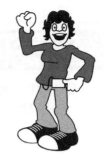

*W*ould *an insulin pump help me prevent complications?*

▼

TIP:

Maybe. If it helps you keep your blood glucose close to normal levels, yes. But an insulin pump is not for everyone. If you have been unable to get your blood glucose levels into goal range, a pump may be a good choice for you. A pump, also called a "continuous subcutaneous insulin infusion system," can do some things that conventional insulin injection therapy can't. Using a pump requires motivation and a willingness to measure your blood sugar several times a day and to make decisions based on the results. A pump cannot "read" your blood sugar, so you will still have to do blood sugar tests regularly to tell the pump how much insulin you need. The downside is the cost. A pump costs about $5,000 to start and about $75 a month to maintain. You should talk to your healthcare team and insurance company about whether a pump would be a good idea for you. Newer pumps have more features and are more reliable than older models. More features allow more flexibility of lifestyle to help you stay in good control.

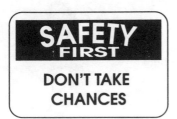

Is it safe for me to use birth control pills if I have diabetes?

▼
TIP:

Oral birth control pills appear to be safe for women with diabetes to take, and they are certainly safer than a pregnancy for which you are unprepared. There is controversy among diabetes specialists about the best form of birth control for women with diabetes. Under certain circumstances, estrogen-containing birth control pills may affect blood sugar and blood cholesterol levels. For this reason, some physicians have not prescribed them for women with diabetes. Studies have shown, however, that blood sugar levels are no different in women who take birth control pills than in women who do not. Similarly, blood cholesterol and lipid levels are no different in diabetic women who use birth control pills than in those who do not. If you are concerned, talk to your health-care team about which method of birth control will work best for you.

*W*ould a successful
pancreas transplant
cure my diabetes?

Bile Duct from Liver

Pancreas

Small Intestine

▼
TIP:

Yes, but a pancreas transplant is not as easy as it sounds. Only a few hospitals in the United States do pancreas transplants. The problem with any transplant is rejection of the foreign tissue by our own bodies. There are drugs that suppress the body's rejection efforts, but these make diabetes control much more difficult. To be considered for a transplant, you have to meet criteria which may vary from center to center:

■ You must have type I diabetes.

■ Most centers will only do a pancreas transplant if you also need a kidney transplant. Anti-rejection drugs are expensive and hazardous, and the kidney transplant would automatically require the same anti-rejection drugs needed for the pancreas transplant.

■ You must have insurance or health coverage to pay for the transplant (many insurance programs consider this an experimental treatment), the medications, and follow-up care needed after the transplant. A pancreas transplant may cost more than $100,000.

Perhaps new therapies will find a way to replace insulin-making cells without requiring anti-rejection medications.

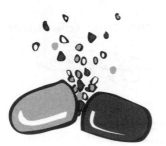

Why are my blood sugars high while I am taking prednisone for my asthma?

▼
TIP:

Prednisone is used for a variety of conditions such as asthma and other lung problems. It acts like a hormone that your body makes called cortisol. Cortisol and prednisone both cause the body to make glucose when you're not eating (like during the night). They can worsen diabetes control. Cortisol is called a stress hormone because the body releases it to deal with stresses like accidents, infections, or burns. That's part of the reason why it takes more insulin to keep blood sugars near normal during an infection. If you have had prednisone prescribed for any reason and you have diabetes, you will need to take more diabetes medication. Prednisone will lose its effect on your blood glucose a day or two after you stop taking it. Your health-care team can help you alter your diabetes treatment until you can stop taking the prednisone.

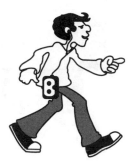

*W*ill *my eleven-year-old son's diabetes have any long-term effects on his psychological health?*

▼
TIP:

Coming to terms with a lifelong, chronic disease like diabetes is a big job for a child. It is not surprising that psychological problems can occur soon after diabetes develops. In general, most children who have family support adapt well and have no long-term psychological problems as a result.

One study has shown that children diagnosed with diabetes between the ages of 8 and 14 were initially more depressed, dependent, and socially withdrawn than other children. By the time a year had passed, most of these problems were gone. By two years after diagnosis, however, children with diabetes again had a higher risk of depression and dependency than children without diabetes.

Children seem to cope with the initial stress of developing diabetes, but as they realize that diabetes is a permanent condition, they may experience a period of depression. It is important for parents to realize this and to contact the health-care team if you are concerned that your child might be depressed. In the interim, be supportive of your child and watchful for signs that might signal the onset of depression, such as a change in appetite, lack of interest in activities, or withdrawal from social groups.

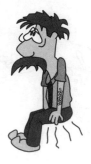

*W**hy do I break out in an itchy rash after my insulin injections?*

▼
TIP:

The rash may be a symptom of an insulin allergy. You may be one of the few people who have to deal with this additional aspect of your diabetes. Although these reactions are becoming more rare with the increasing use of human insulin, up to 2% of all people with diabetes will experience some form of allergy to their injected insulin. Most insulin allergies go away on their own within the first year of insulin treatment, but some don't. You may not be allergic to all forms of insulin. Your doctor can perform skin tests to determine exactly what kinds of insulin you are most allergic to. If necessary, you can even receive "allergy shots" with very dilute preparations of insulin to desensitize you to the allergic effects of insulin.

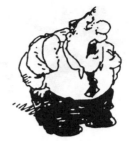

*W*hy should I check my sugar when I can "feel" when it's high or low?

▼
TIP:

B ecause you can't always feel it. Many people with diabetes believe that they have specific feelings when their sugar is either too high or too low. Although this may occasionally be true, it is unreliable. Studies have been done in people with diabetes in which their blood sugar has been acutely raised or lowered without them knowing which. They were then asked what they thought their blood sugar level was. No individual could accurately predict when his or her blood sugar was high and how high it was. On the other hand, many people could tell when their blood sugar was low or at least dropping rapidly. Unfortunately, when you consistently have high blood sugar, you often feel like your blood sugar is low even when it is still high. Because you make important decisions depending on your blood sugar level, check your blood sugar before taking insulin, exercising, or driving a car.

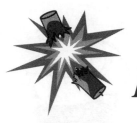

*H*ow can the sugar in my blood be
harmful when it's so common in food?

Sugar

▼
TIP:

The sugar in food is powerful. It can be thought of as tiny packets of bundled up energy. Normally, the body does not let the amount of sugar in the blood rise very high because it will react with the wrong tissues. In fact, of all the substances that circulate in your blood, sugar is one the body regulates most carefully. Even in people without diabetes, too much sugar is thought to be responsible for many of the changes that occur with aging. However, when a person has diabetes, his or her body cannot prevent high blood glucose levels from occurring. Over long periods of time, high levels of sugar can cause serious damage to many tissues, especially your eyes, kidneys, and nerves. This damage results in the "complications" of diabetes. These can be avoided or greatly delayed by leading a healthy lifestyle and keeping your blood sugar in your goal range.

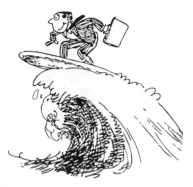

*S*hould I expect my blood sugars to level off after I start a new diabetes medicine?

▼
TIP:

Yes. Blood sugars initially fall in response to the medicine. But there is an effect that has to do with the fact that high blood sugars tend to cause more high blood sugars. If your blood sugar has been high for some time, your pancreas can't immediately readjust. Your body has been using insulin poorly. When you interrupt the cycle and spend more time in the normal blood sugar range, you begin to increase your body's ability to stay there. After several weeks of improved control, many patients find that they need less insulin or oral medication to keep their blood sugars under control. It may take more medication to get your blood sugars to begin to go down, but how much medicine you need may decrease as your overall diabetes control improves.

Some patients with type II diabetes who take a diabetes medication and who also start exercising and eating better find that, after a while, they can stop their medication as long as they continue the other activities. Talk to your health-care team before stopping any medication. If you get the "go ahead," monitor your blood sugars while you continue with your diet and exercise programs. However, at the first sign that your blood sugar levels are going back up, contact your team.

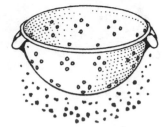

Why did my weight increase after I got my blood sugars under better control?

▼
TIP:

Some oral diabetes medications, such as glipizide and glyburide, and insulin will tend to cause weight gain when you achieve better sugar control. You are having a very common experience. When your blood sugars were high, you were wasting many calories in your urine. The kidneys can only absorb a limited amount of sugar and then, like a sieve, they let the extra sugar go through into the urine. This loss of sugar in the urine begins at a blood sugar level of about 200 mg/dl. So you waste part of the calories you are eating when your blood sugar exceeds this level. This may sound like a great way to eat too much and also control your weight, but the long-term effect of high sugar is very damaging to many parts of your body. Your body needs insulin to store amino acids (the building blocks of protein in muscle) and to make muscle. So, take your medication as prescribed by your health-care team, reduce your food intake, and exercise regularly to control your weight.

Chapter Three:
HEALTH FOODS

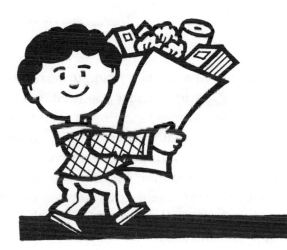

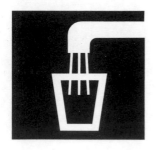

Will chromium help me stay healthy and improve my blood sugar control?

▼
TIP:

Your body does need some chromium to be healthy, but you're probably asking whether you need to take a chromium supplement. Most people do not need these supplements. Chromium is a naturally occurring mineral found in tap water and also present in tiny amounts in our bodies. Whether or not taking chromium will help you has been examined in many research studies. If you're getting enough chromium in your diet, there is no need for additional vitamin and mineral supplementation for the majority of people with diabetes. Adequate diet means that you are getting a normal amount of calories from a variety of foods. Most people get into trouble when they eliminate one or more of the food groups or drastically reduce the calories needed to maintain a reasonable weight.

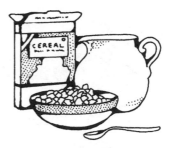

*W*ill fiber in my diet help me?

▼
TIP:

High fiber diets may be beneficial to you, particularly if you have high blood fats or impaired glucose tolerance. Fiber is found primarily in fruits, vegetables, beans, and cereals such as wheat and oats. Insoluble fibers like cellulose, found in wheat bran and celery, are dense and chewy. Soluble fibers, in whole oats and green peas, are soft and rather gel-like when mixed with water. Most fiber is not absorbed by the body, so it passes out in the stool. Any compounds that are bound by fiber in the intestine are also not absorbed. Many studies have been done to determine if fiber is beneficial. Most studies show a positive (although limited) effect on blood fats. That's why high fiber diets usually lower blood cholesterol. Some studies (primarily in type II diabetes) have also shown an improvement in blood sugar levels, but this improvement is usually small. The easiest way to increase the fiber in your diet is to take a tablespoon of pseudophilin (Metamucil®) before you go to sleep. Also, you can eat more whole grains for breakfast, such as oatmeal or branflakes.

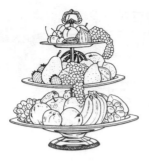

*S*hould I use fructose as a sweetener when I bake?

▼
TIP:

Fructose is not necessarily better for you than plain sugar. Fructose is a naturally occurring sweetener like table sugar (sucrose). It may produce a smaller rise in blood sugar than the same number of calories of table sugar. This is good for people with diabetes; however, large amounts of fructose can increase your total cholesterol and bad cholesterol (LDL) levels. That's why fructose is really no better for you than sugar. People with abnormal blood cholesterol levels should avoid consuming large amounts of fructose.

W̶ill ginseng help me control my blood sugar?

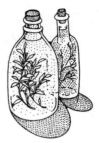

▼
TIP:

Ginseng, derived from plants, is a chemical that has been used for many centuries to improve overall health and increase energy and well being. It is often made into tea and taken with food. It is very popular here and in some European and Eastern countries. There are very few studies which test its beneficial effects in people with diabetes. Recently, one small short-term study from Finland suggested that individuals with type II diabetes who drink ginseng tea daily may have a lower blood sugar than those who do not. Whether or not this effect lasts longer than one year is not known. At this time, ginseng is not a recommended treatment for diabetes, but that recommendation could change. Stay in touch with your health-care team for updates.

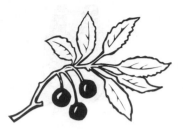

A re there any useful herbal remedies for diabetes?

▼
TIP:

We don't know. Diet or herbal remedies were all we had for most of the 2,000 years since diabetes was first described. Health food stores carry dozens of products designed for people with diabetes to use, ranging from blueberry leaf and wild cherry bark to preparations called "Hysugar" and "Losugar." Few of these products have been tested or proven to be safe and effective. Because herbal remedies are classified as food supplements, they are not regulated by the Food and Drug Administration. Moreover, none of these products alone result in adequate blood sugar control in most people with diabetes. You should discuss any anti-diabetes health food products with your health-care team. You may find that they are somewhat skeptical, but they will probably not object to the use of these products in moderation if you are demonstrating good control of your diabetes and doing the other things necessary to stay healthy with diabetes.

W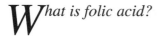

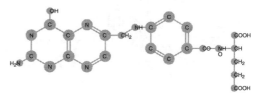

▼
TIP:

F olic acid (or folate) is a member of the B vitamin family found in green, leafy vegetables. It plays an important role in several chemical processes in your body. Many medical experts are currently recommending increased intake of folic acid because folic acid lowers homocysteine levels in our bodies. Homocysteine is a byproduct of the metabolic break-down of a particular amino acid (the building blocks of pro-teins) called cysteine. There is a growing amount of scientific evidence which suggests that people with high levels of homocysteine are more likely to suffer from a heart attack or stroke. Although the issue remains to be settled, some studies suggest that people with diabetes have higher than normal amounts of homocysteine in their bodies, and this fact may be related to the increased number of heart attacks and strokes that occur in people with diabetes. Thus, it may be beneficial for people with diabetes to supplement their diet with the Recommended Daily Allowance (RDA) of 180–200 micro-grams per day for men and women and 400 micrograms for pregnant women. This is the amount of folic acid usually found in daily multivitamin preparations.

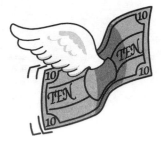

*W*ill magnesium supplements help
my diabetes?

▼
TIP:

Probably not. The American Diabetes Association does not
recommend routine blood tests for magnesium levels, nor
does it recommend that people take magnesium unless they
have been shown to be deficient in this mineral. Magnesium
deficiency may play a role in causing insulin resistance, carbohydrate intolerance, and high blood pressure. People who eat a
varied diet should not become magnesium deficient because
magnesium is found in many foods (including cereals, nuts,
and green vegetables).

People at risk of magnesium deficiency are those with
congestive heart failure, potassium or calcium deficiency, and
those who are pregnant. Others at risk have had heart attacks,
ketoacidosis, long-term feeding through the veins, long-term
alcohol abuse, or have taken drugs such as diuretics over long
periods of time. If a blood test shows these people need
magnesium, a supplement may be given by the doctor. People
with kidney disease should be very careful not to get too much
magnesium and only take it under a doctor's care.

Pineal Gland

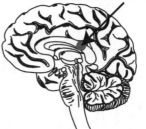

*I*s the melatonin miracle real?

▼
TIP:

Melatonin is a substance that is normally secreted by a small part of the brain called the pineal gland. The exact role that it plays in humans is not clear, but research suggests that it may help regulate your sleep. It has become popular and is sold in health food stores. Many unproven beneficial effects have been attributed to melatonin, including better sleep, elimination of jet lag, reversal of the aging process, enhancement of sex, and protection against disease. Are these claims too good to be true? Yes. There is very little scientific proof that melatonin is beneficial. If you buy melatonin, you are probably just wasting your money. You may ask, "Is there any harm if I take melatonin for sleep?" The problem is that there are no long-term studies which show that melatonin is safe. In fact, some doctors fear permanent damage to your normal sleep patterns if you take melatonin. There may also be other hazards that will become known only after melatonin has been in use several more years. For now, it is wise not to take melatonin supplements until there is better evidence to support its safety and effectiveness.

Chapter Four:
DIETARY ADVICE

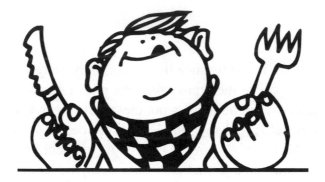

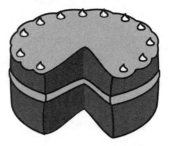

*H*ow can I overcome my craving
for chocolate?

▼
TIP:

Give in once in a while! By denying your desire for chocolate (or any other particular food), you are setting yourself
up for failure. If you find yourself craving a food and having to
put effort into avoiding it, you may eventually give in and eat
too much of it. Then your blood sugar control suffers and you
feel guilty and depressed. Plan on some healthy ways to satisfy
yourself. For chocolate lovers, dark or bitter chocolate is preferred to milk chocolate that has higher dairy fat. We suggest
low-fat frozen yogurt. It tastes great, has less than 1 gram of
fat, and is inexpensive. Another treat is chocolate graham
crackers, which may also be used for making desserts. Make a
fancy dessert with angel food cake, strawberries, and chocolate
syrup. Yes, the syrup has some sugar in it but it is almost fat
free. Whether you have type I or type II diabetes, fat must be a
concern for you and is actually the worst part of most candies.
Recent research has shown us that sugar has about the same
effect as an equal amount of potatoes or rice on your blood
sugar. If you can find some relatively low-fat foods that fit into
your diet plan, go for it.

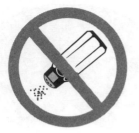

What diet change must I make to improve my blood pressure?

▼
TIP:

Lowering the sodium in your diet may make a big difference in your blood pressure if you are sensitive to sodium. Less sodium in your body means you will retain less water. There will be less fluid in your blood vessels, and less "pressure" in the system. Sodium is a major part of table salt. Sodium is also used as a preservative and flavor enhancer in foods that may not even taste "salty." Try these tips to lower your sodium intake: 1) Always taste your food before reaching for the salt shaker. 2) Use pepper and other seasonings to add flavor before adding salt. 3) Cook with a variety of seasonings, such as onion and garlic. 4) Add a dash of lemon juice to vegetables and salads to brighten the flavor. 5) Avoid "seasoned salt" or garlic salt: use garlic powder or fresh garlic. 6) Try a commercial salt-free seasoning mix and carry a small container with you. 7) Ask for foods to be prepared without salt in restaurants and ask for sauces "on the side." 8) Read the labels on prepared foods and canned goods to find the high salt items and look for "no salt added" or lower sodium products. Remember, the closer to nature a food is, the more likely it will be low in salt.

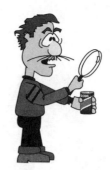

D oes reading food labels help me stay healthy?

▼
TIP:

Yes. It gives you important information that can help you eat healthy meals and snacks. New regulations by the Food and Drug Administration have increased the information that must be put on food labels. Food labels must include:

1) The standard serving size

2) Calories and calories from fat per serving

3) A list of nutrients and ingredients

4) The recommended daily amounts of nutrients in the food

5) The relationship between the food and any disease it may affect.

Try to make a habit of reading the labels of the foods you buy and become familiar with the amount of calories, fat, carbohydrate, and sodium in them. For many foods, you will have a choice of different brand names, and by comparing the information on the labels, you can choose the brand that is healthier. Food label information helps you keep track of the amount of nutrients you are eating daily. This information is vital to a healthy diet.

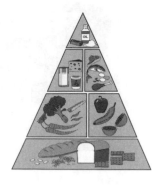

*W*ill the new *"Food Guide Pyramid"* help me live healthier with diabetes?

▼
TIP:

Yes. The food guide pyramid was developed as a guide for all Americans to healthy eating. It's healthy eating for people with diabetes, too. The pyramid shape is used to tell you how much to eat of different foods. The bottom section is the largest section. It is the bread, cereal, rice, and pasta group and most people should eat 6 to 11 servings a day. The two sections above the starches are the vegetable group (3–5 servings a day) and the fruit group (2–4 servings a day). You will notice that these first three sections together cover more than half of the pyramid. This tells you that half or more of your daily food intake should come from these foods. The next two sections are the dairy (2–3 servings a day) and the meat, poultry, and fish group (2–3 servings a day). You don't need as much of these foods. Also, they may be high in fat. The small top section contains the fats, oils, and sweets group. You need very little of these foods, which is why they don't have serving suggestions. They can be very high in calories without much nutrition. Following the food guide pyramid can be an easy and healthy way for the person with diabetes to achieve good health and nutrition.

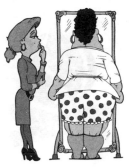

*S*hould I join an expensive diet/weight
reduction program to lose weight?

▼
TIP:

We don't recommend it. You will probably waste your time and your money. Advertisements for these programs usually show "before" and "after" photographs of heavy people who have lost weight. What these advertisements don't show you are the people who never lost a pound. More importantly, long-term studies have shown that almost all of the people who lose weight rapidly over several months gain it all back by the end of five years. This has also been the experience of our patients who have tried these programs. Also, very-low-calorie diets can be dangerous, as chemical imbalances and vitamin deficiencies can occur. A much better plan to lose weight is to make a small change in your lifestyle so that you lose only one half to one pound per month. Over five years, this small change equals a 50 pound weight loss! In comparison to expensive diet programs, low cost weight reduction programs such as Weight Watchers or TOPS (Take Off Pounds Sensibly) can provide much support and advice for you. In addition, your health-care team can be of great help in suggesting ways of making small but positive changes in your lifestyle to accomplish your weight goals.

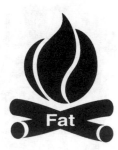

*W*hy *do I spill ketones in my urine?*

▼
TIP:

K etones in the urine show that fat is being used for fuel by your body. This typically occurs: (1) when you do not have enough insulin in your body to metabolize sugar as fuel, or (2) when you are fasting. Thus, spilling ketones into your urine means either that your body is dangerously low on insulin or that your diet is working. When ketones build up due to a lack of insulin, the condition is called ketoacidosis, and it can be dangerous. Ketoacidosis is more common in type I diabetes, occurring when people are first diagnosed with diabetes, when they stop taking insulin for some reason, or when they are ill. Most people develop symptoms that make them consult a doctor, such as stomach pain, nausea or vomiting, rapid breathing, frequent urination, extreme thirst, or fatigue.

If you are on a diet that does not provide enough calories to your body, then your body burns fat for energy. This is the effect you want from your diet, because burning fat will cause you to lose weight. A by-product of fat metabolism, however, is ketones, and these ketones spill into your urine just as they do in ketoacidosis. If you are feeling fine and controlling your blood sugar, then the ketones in your urine are probably a safe result of your diet.

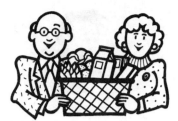

How can I get my husband to follow his diabetic diet?

▼
TIP:

We have several suggestions. There are many reasons that your husband might not follow his prescribed diet. First, he may not understand the meal plan. Did your husband see a registered dietitian (RD) and receive easily understood written instructions describing his diet? Second, your husband may not believe that the diet will work. Ask him to try the prescribed diet for one month and measure his weight and blood sugar daily to see what the effects are. Then he can decide if the diet will help him achieve his goals. Third, your husband may not want to eat foods that are "different" from those that the rest of the family eats. It helps if the whole family changes to a healthier diet. (A "diabetic" diet is the same balanced healthy diet that everyone should eat.) The RD can help him fit some of his favorite foods into the meal plan. Fourth, do you understand the details of the diet? If you select and prepare the food that your husband eats, you may want to discuss the diet with the health-care team's dietitian. Finally, remember that changing eating habits will involve a change in lifestyle, which is difficult for anyone. Your husband will need support, understanding, and patience to achieve his goals.

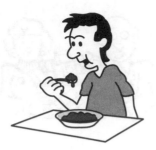

*I*s it a good idea to eat 4 or 5 small meals during the day instead of 3 large meals?

▼
TIP:

Yes! Scientists have been looking for the ideal frequency of meals since the beginning of diabetes research. There are many benefits to eating small amounts of food over the course of the day instead of in larger amounts at meal times. These benefits include decreased blood sugar levels after a meal, reduced insulin requirements over the course of the day, and decreased blood cholesterol levels. These benefits probably stem from a slow, continuous absorption of food from your gut, which spares your body the work of switching over to a "fasting" state. Also, eating several small meals a day may decrease your hunger and reduce the number of calories you eat during the day. Most studies have investigated the effect of eating six to eight meals a day. Finally, there are diabetes medications available, such as acarbose, which slow the absorption of food and have much the same effect as eating your food slowly over the course of the day. The practice of nibbling is not for everyone; but if you are able to maintain good blood sugar control and a desirable body weight doing it, then continue.

*H*ow can I use the waist/hip
ratio to improve my health?

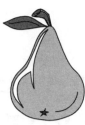
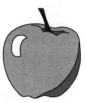

Good Shape   **Bad Shape**

▼
TIP:

The waist/hip ratio can be used to predict your risk of
developing heart disease in the future. Take a tape measure
and measure the circumference of your body at its largest
diameter at the level of your hips. Next, measure the size of
your waist (your stomach) at its largest diameter. Be honest,
don't pull in your stomach when measuring. OK, now you are
ready. Divide your waist size in inches by your hip size in
inches. If the answer is less than 1.0 for men (0.85 for
women), then your shape is good. What this means is that your
body is pear-shaped rather than apple-shaped. If the result is
more than 1.0 for men (0.85 for women), you are at an
increased risk to develop heart disease. The reason for the
increased risk is that you have more fat in the stomach area
than on your hips and thighs. For unknown reasons, fat located
above the hips is a major risk factor for future heart disease. If
you are at an increased risk, you need to work on losing
weight. After you have lost 5 lbs., remeasure your waist/hip
ratio. Keep reducing your weight until your waist/hip ratio is
below 1.0 if you are a man (0.85 if you are a woman). All obesity is bad for your health, but obesity above your waist is
especially hazardous.

Chapter Five:
COMPLICATIONS—MICRO*

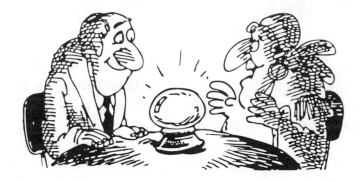

*disease of the small blood vessels

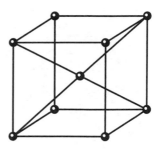

*W*hat does the term A.G.E. mean
in reference to diabetes?

▼
TIP:

ood question! A.G.E. is an abbreviation for Advanced
Glycosylation End products. This complicated name
describes the process of sugar becoming permanently attached
to body tissues. The sugar may cause damage so that the tissues can no longer carry out their normal function.

A common example is glycosylated hemoglobin, which is
glucose permanently attached to hemoglobin protein in your
red blood cells. However, since new red blood cells are
continuously made by your body, little long-term damage
results from this attached glucose. In contrast, tissues in your
eyes, kidneys, and nerves remain in your body for a long period
of time so that the attached sugar can do significant damage.

A new medicine called aminoguanidine can block sugar
from permanently attaching to and damaging your body
tissues. Hopefully, this medicine will prevent some of the
complications of diabetes. This medicine is currently being
tested in many medical centers throughout the United States.
Studies in animals suggest it should work well in humans. If it
does, then many of the complications of diabetes will be
preventable.

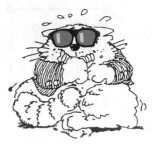

W̶hat kinds of eye problems are caused by diabetes?

▼
TIP:

Diabetes is the number one cause of blindness in the United States. Fortunately, many eye problems are treatable if they are identified early. One of the most serious eye problems caused by diabetes is retinopathy. In this disease fragile blood vessels grow in the back of the eye and can bleed easily. Such bleeding can cloud the vision and lead to permanent scarring of the back of the eye (the retina). People with diabetes also have cataracts (a permanent clouding of the lens), "floaters" which temporarily interfere with vision, and a swelling of the eye nerves which can cause permanent damage to your sight (macular edema). Abnormal function of the nerves which control the eye muscles can result in double vision. All people who develop double vision should see an eye doctor as soon as possible to rule out other possible causes, such as a small stroke. Cataracts can be corrected surgically. Laser therapy helps stop retinopathy or macular edema if it is performed before there is too much damage. A yearly eye examination by a doctor who specializes in diabetic eye disease is the best way to detect eye problems in the early stages and keeping your blood sugar near normal can help reduce your risk of eye disease.

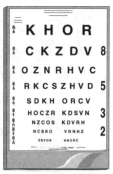

*W**hy would my health-care team be concerned about my becoming pregnant if I have high blood pressure and have had laser treatment of my eye problems?*

▼
TIP:

M any changes in blood flow and pressure occur during pregnancy that can aggravate eye disease and kidney disease. The number of blood pressure medications that can be used safely during pregnancy and not injure a developing fetus are limited. You should discuss the options and the severity of your complications openly with your health-care team as part of your pregnancy planning process. Existing complications of diabetes can worsen during pregnancy. This is not to say that you should not get pregnant if you have mild diabetic complications. Many women with long-standing diabetes are able to have a normal pregnancy. However, the complications may make the pregnancy more difficult. One means of assessing the risks of pregnancy is called the "White classification" and is used by some obstetricians specializing in patients with diabetes and pregnancy. How long you have had diabetes and the severity of your complications determine the level of risk using the White classification.

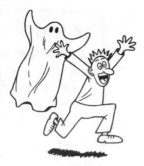

*C*an I ignore the risks of diabetic complications since the thought of them scares me?

▼
TIP:

No, because there are some things you can do now to prevent the disabling complications of diabetes. Adjusting your food, physical activity, and medication (if any) to bring your blood glucose levels to near normal ranges can help you avoid or delay complications. Research has proven that. You express emotions that most of us go through at some time in our lives. All of us have fears of growing old or disabled, whether we have diabetes or not. The challenge we all face is to live healthy; we want to live well every day that we live. We want to be fully functional and independent. You can decide to ignore the changes taking place in your body but that won't make them go away. Or you can take charge to change the outcome so that you can live your life without fear. Your knowledge of the effects of diabetic complications on your body is information that can give you power over the future!

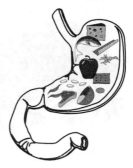

*D*uring a meal, why do I get filled up
before I finish eating?

▼
TIP:

You may have a complication of diabetes causing your
symptoms that is called "diabetic gastroparesis." It means
that the stomach empties very slowly. It is caused by damage
to the nerves that control the pace at which food leaves the
stomach and gets processed in the gut. Some people experience nausea, while others may only note that they can't eat as
much at one time. If the rate of food emptying from your
stomach is too slow and you took insulin before the meal, your
blood sugar may fall before the food has had a chance to be
absorbed. You may have to take your insulin injection right at
the time of the meal to prevent low blood sugars and to match
the absorption of your carbohydrate. High-fiber or high-fat
foods tend to make gastroparesis worse. There are some medications which can help improve gut function. Talk to your
health-care team about the best approach for you.

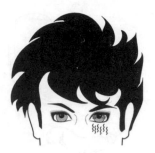

Could my diabetes cause one of my eyes to be red and painful?

▼
TIP:

Perhaps. Allergies to pollens and dust in the air are the most common cause of red eyes, but this rarely causes pain. An eye infection which can cause red eyes is viral conjunctivitis, or "pink eye". Unfortunately, this infection has to run its course because antibiotics cannot help speed recovery. Serious bacterial infections can start on the surface or behind the eye of a person with diabetes and require strong antibiotics to cure. A common complaint of patients with either viral or bacterial infections is that they wake up in the morning with their eyelashes sticking together from the pus that has collected over the night. If your pain is more like a pressure sensation, then you may have glaucoma. Glaucoma is too much pressure in the eye and is more common in people with diabetes. It can be detected during your yearly eye exam. The test involves blowing a small puff of air (which doesn't hurt) at the surface of the eye. Your doctor may prescribe eye drops that lower the pressure in the eye. This condition is definitely worth finding early because it is treatable. Left untreated, glaucoma can result in blindness.

*W*ill my diabetic kidney disease get worse if I get pregnant?

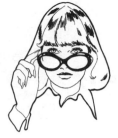

▼
TIP:

There is about a 30% chance that your kidney function will worsen during pregnancy, but these changes often improve after delivery of the infant. Many people with diabetes will first show signs of abnormal kidney function (spilling of protein in the urine) during pregnancy. If you have kidney disease before getting pregnant, then there is a chance that it will get worse during pregnancy.

Moreover, babies born to mothers with diabetic kidney disease have a higher risk of stillbirth, respiratory distress, jaundice, and abnormally small body size compared to babies of diabetic mothers without kidney problems. Also, about 30% of these babies are born prematurely. You will need to have tight blood sugar control and careful control of blood pressure during pregnancy. Thus, it can be done, but you should know the risk before you get pregnant.

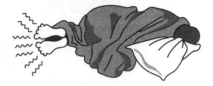

Why do my feet burn at night when I'm trying to go to sleep?

▼
TIP:

The nerves in your feet have been affected by your diabetes. "Painful neuropathy" is a term used to describe diabetic feet that are painful without an obvious cause. People with painful neuropathy usually describe a "pins and needles" sensation or a dull burning in the feet and legs which is more apparent at night (when there are few other things to distract you). You may also experience frequent leg cramps. Since painful neuropathy is difficult to cure once it is established, the best treatment is to prevent it by controlling your blood sugar. These nerve problems occur more frequently in men, in individuals who have had diabetes for many years, are tall, smoke, or have poor blood sugar control.

If you already have painful neuropathy, there are treatments available that provide some relief for about 50% of people. These treatments include the use of antidepressant medicines, certain heart medications, and creams made from chili peppers (capsaicin). These creams are rubbed on the feet to desensitize them. If you do not get relief from one of these treatments, the good news is that the pain from this neuropathy often lessens over time.

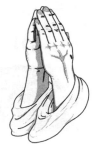

*I*s there a simple test to see whether my
diabetes is causing my hands to be stiff
and rigid?

▼
TIP:

High blood sugars over a long period of time can increase
the stiffness of tissue around your finger joints. This can
eventually cause stiff hands and prevent you from straighten-
ing your fingers. This stiffness may make it difficult to write or
to pick up small items and do other fine movements. An easy
test for this condition is called the "prayer sign" in which you
hold your hands together, one palm facing the other palm, to
see whether your fingers can lie flat against each other. If a
space exists between your right and left hands when your
hands are pushed together (as in the above figure), this is a
"positive" prayer sign. High sugars may be causing this condition. Arthritis can also cause a "positive" prayer sign. In the
near future, new medications may become available which will
reduce this stiffness. In the meantime, you should try to keep
your blood sugars as close to your goal range as possible.

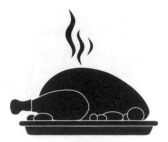

Should I eat more protein to replace the protein I am losing in my urine?

▼
TIP:

Usually the answer is no. The protein that you are losing in your urine (known as "spilling protein") is a sign that the filters in your kidney are showing wear and tear. Normally, the blood in your body goes through your kidneys to remove waste products. Kidneys act like a sieve which retains valuable chemicals but lets water go through. The protein in your blood is supposed to stay in your body, but when the kidney filters are damaged from years of high blood sugar and high blood pressure, they let protein slip through as well. Plus the waste products from protein can be stressful to the kidney.

Reducing the amount of protein in your diet helps the kidneys and may slow damage to them. You should talk to your health-care team about reducing protein in your diet. You might not know that many foods such as cereals and grains contain protein. You may need help designing a diet plan that helps you reduce overall protein but gives you the essential types and amounts that you need. Wise food choices and following your meal plan are an important part of keeping your kidneys healthy.

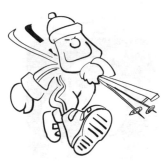

Should I limit my exercise program for one month after laser therapy on my eyes?

▼
TIP:

Yes. Diabetic eye disease (retinopathy) is a condition of overgrowth of fragile blood vessels in the eye that can cause bleeding, scarring, and loss of vision if they break. Even though you have had laser therapy, you should still be careful to avoid situations that can stress these vessels. Avoid exercises that cause you to strain, such as weight lifting or any exercise that causes you to hold your breath. Underwater diving can also cause increased pressure in the eye and should be avoided. Another consequence of laser therapy is the possibility of a loss in peripheral vision (the ability to see clearly off to the side). For this reason, some sports (such as racquetball or tennis) may be hazardous, since they require you to respond to a ball coming at a high speed from all angles. You should discuss any exercise program with your eye doctor if you have had laser therapy.

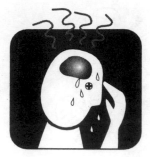

Why have I recently begun to sweat profusely when I sit down and eat food, even though the food does not contain hot, spicy items?

▼
TIP:

A complication of diabetes which is related to nerve damage is called "gustatory sweating." The person with diabetes breaks out in a sweat from chewing food. The cause of this sweating is not known, but it may be related to having high blood sugars for a long time. You may also have increased sweating or flushing of the neck and chest. Cheese or chocolate are the most common foods to cause sweating, but pickles, alcohol, vinegar, fresh fruits, and salty foods may do it, too. Various types of medications have been tried to treat this problem with varying levels of success. Although in some cases it stops by itself, keeping your blood sugar as normal as possible and avoiding specific foods may prevent sweating caused by food.

Chapter Six:
COMPLICATIONS—MACRO*

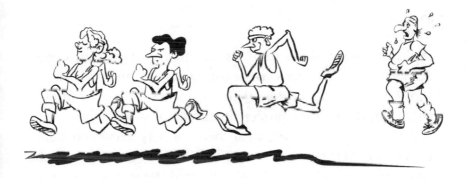

*disease of the large blood vessels

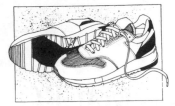

Since I don't want to end up with foot problems, how do I know if my athletic shoes are okay?

TIP:

It is best to buy shoes from a store that has experienced personnel who know how to measure your feet and fit your shoes correctly. A Certified Pedorthist is a specialist in fitting shoes and inserts for a proper fit with no pressure points. When you get new shoes, wear them for only a few hours and then check your feet for any red areas or sore places where the shoes might be rubbing. Even well-fitted shoes may have a seam or area that rubs on your foot. Get padded athletic socks that protect your feet from blisters. Athletic shoes have become very high-tech these days and have different features depending on the exercise you are planning to do. It is a good idea to get the ones with extra cushion because this reduces the wear and tear on your joints. Look in the Yellow Pages for stores that specialize in athletic shoes.

*A*m I at more risk to develop heart
disease because I have diabetes?

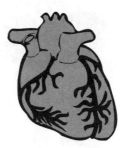

▼
TIP:

Yes. For unknown reasons, having diabetes does put you at
an increased risk of heart disease and other diseases that
are caused by blocked arteries. That is why it is very important
for you to minimize your other risk factors by getting plenty of
exercise, keeping your weight normal, avoiding cholesterol
and fatty foods (saturated fat), and maintaining normal blood
pressure. Walking is a good exercise and helps in all those
areas as well as reducing stress. Most important (at least in our
opinion) is that you do not smoke cigarettes. If you are already
smoking, join a "quit smoking" support group available in
most communities and health-care facilities. Nicotine skin
patches may help. Many of the risk factors that cause heart
disease can be greatly reduced with a healthy lifestyle, and this
should be your goal with or without diabetes. However, since
you already have one risk factor for heart disease (diabetes),
there is even more reason to reduce other risk factors.

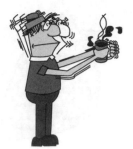

*W*hy do I get dizzy when I stand up?

▼
TIP:

Patients with long-standing diabetes can lose the ability to vary their blood pressure in response to changes in posture. A drop in blood pressure when you stand up can cause dizziness, temporary loss of vision, or fainting spells.

You may be experiencing "postural dizziness," which can be serious. Abnormal function of the nerves that regulate your heart and blood vessels is the most common cause of postural dizziness, but other causes must be ruled out by your health-care team. Blood pressure medications, such as diuretics, can cause postural dizziness as can antidepressants, nitroglycerine, and certain calcium-blocking drugs.

If your postural dizziness is due to diabetes alone, then you will require specific treatment for this problem. Tilting your bed so that the head is 6–9 inches higher than the foot may reduce your dizziness. Other therapies include carefully increasing the salt in your diet, wearing support stockings to prevent blood from pooling in your legs, or taking a hormone pill (Florinef®) to help your body retain fluid. These treatments can be dangerous in people who have heart disease, so be sure to consult your health-care team before trying any of them.

*I*s my 25 years of diabetes to blame for
my recent trouble maintaining erections?

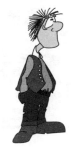

▼
TIP:

Maybe, but there are other causes. Your doctor should
begin with psychological and emotional causes. This
includes questions about depression, because depression affects
sex drive. Other causes may be poor circulation to the penis or
hormone levels. Blood flow to the penis may be too low to get
or maintain erections. Long-term high blood sugars can affect
these blood vessels or the nerves to the penis. If this is the
problem, there are devices to aid you in getting an erection. All
men have reduced male hormone levels as they get older.
Replacing these hormones with monthly injections (or daily
skin patches) of testosterone, may improve sex drive. There is
an oral medication that may help maintain erections (yohimbine), and recently an injection into the penis was developed to
help sustain erections. As a side effect, some medicines can
cause sexual problems, and switching from one to another may
help. Drinking alcohol can affect male hormone levels and can
depress your brain's ability to get sexually aroused. There are
many causes and many treatments. See your health-care team
for an evaluation or referral to a specialist.

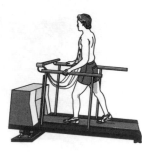

Should I have a yearly test to see if I have heart disease?

▼
TIP:

A sk your diabetes-care team each year if you have any health complaints that would indicate that a heart test is necessary. Heart disease is the cause of death in about 80% of people with diabetes. People with diabetes do not always develop symptoms (such as chest pain) when they are having heart stress or even a heart attack, and heart disease can occur at a young age. Testing is required to diagnose heart disease at a stage when it is treatable. If you have had diabetes for many years, consult your health-care team to see if a screening test for silent heart disease is necessary—especially if you plan to start an exercise program or you have multiple risks for developing heart disease. Your health-care team will probably refer you to a heart doctor (cardiologist) for these tests, and the type of test may vary. Some cardiologists prefer a simple exercise treadmill test, where your heart is monitored while you walk uphill on a treadmill. Many cardiologists now prefer to stress your heart with a medication instead of exercise. A test, called a dipyridamole stress test, shows how your heart functions when it works hard and may reveal areas of heart damage. This damage may then be treated with medications or surgery.

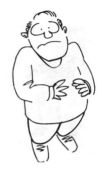

*S*ince I can't reach or see my toes very well, how can I adequately care for my feet?

▼
TIP:

Many people with diabetes have difficulty seeing their feet well and trimming their toenails. The reasons for this problem are many, including poor eyesight, obesity, arthritis, back pain, and other medical conditions that may prevent leaning over toward the floor. Have a member of your family examine your feet once a day for sores and nail problems. We strongly recommend that most people with diabetes not try to cut their own toenails, but go regularly to a podiatrist for routine foot care. Podiatrists are trained to provide good foot hygiene and nail care. They can be located in the Yellow Pages under Physicians & Surgeons, D.P.M. (Podiatric), or ask your health-care team for a referral. Good foot care is extremely important to good health. It may save your feet.

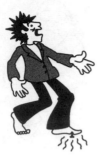

*D*o I need to have special foot care if my feet don't hurt?

▼
TIP:

Yes. If you have had diabetes for many years, it is common not to feel pain in your feet. Thus you may not notice sores and blisters that would normally cause you to avoid walking. Even if you don't have any sores, corns, callouses, or thickened toenails, you should still check your feet daily and use a moisturizing lotion after bathing—but not between your toes. Going barefoot is not recommended because of injuries to bare feet. Always take off your shoes and socks during your quarterly visit to the health-care team as a reminder to have your feet checked. The team will test to see if you can feel a soft touch or little changes of direction in your toes, as well as examining your reflexes and your ability to feel a tuning fork vibration. They will look for areas of skin breakdown on the bottom of your feet and between your toes, and will check to be sure that you do not have an ingrown toenail. Ingrown nails easily become infected and require special care. You should see a podiatrist (DPM) if you have a tendency to develop ingrown toenails. A podiatrist will also remove any callouses you have. Many of the infections that end in leg amputation started out as tiny, nonpainful foot sores that didn't heal.

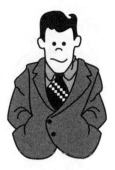

*W*hy *did my doctor start me on a cholesterol lowering drug even though my cholesterol levels are only borderline high?*

▼
TIP:

B ecause he wants to prevent or delay heart disease. Heart disease is the number one cause of death in people with diabetes. Blood lipid (or fat) levels are one of the most important ways to determine your risk for developing heart disease. People with diabetes tend to develop heart disease with lower lipid levels than nondiabetic patients, so some doctors try early on to lower blood lipid levels in their diabetic patients. This is probably a good idea, especially if you are a person who has several other risk factors for the development of heart disease. These risk factors include smoking, high blood pressure, and a history of heart disease at a young age among your close family members.

Because the risk of heart disease is high among all people with diabetes, they should stop smoking, eat a low-fat, low-cholesterol diet, avoid weight gain, and exercise regularly. If these measures fail, then drug therapy is usually considered.

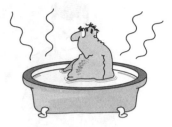

If I am on insulin, is it all right for me to sit in a hot tub?

▼
TIP:

U nder certain conditions. People with diabetes should be careful with hot tubs or saunas. Excessive heat can make the heart beat faster and if you have an underlying heart problem (like angina), you may end up with serious heart damage. When your whole body gets overheated, your heart tries to increase the blood flow to your skin to get rid of some of the extra heat you have absorbed from the water or steam. If you use insulin to control your diabetes, you may find that this increased blood flow to the fat (where you inject your insulin) increases the rate at which the insulin is absorbed. So a dose of a longer-acting insulin that is intended to last throughout the night will be absorbed much more rapidly. This causes low blood sugars during the hours after you get out of the tub. We recommend temperatures no higher than 105 degrees and that you stay in the water for no longer than twenty minutes. Discuss your plans with your health-care team.

*W*hy do I sometimes leak urine?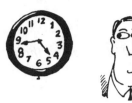

▼
TIP:

Approximately 25% of all people with long-term diabetes have some problems with bladder function. Most of these problems result from faulty signals from the nerves that control the bladder. Some of these problems are minor, such as an inability to completely empty your bladder when you urinate, a slow rate of urine flow, or an inability to tell when your bladder is full until it is overflowing. When you accidentally leak urine, the problem is usually more advanced and is called incontinence. The most common cause of incontinence is an inability to tell whether your bladder is full, so the bladder becomes too full and overflows. Men with incontinence often have a large prostate gland that can be treated with medicine or corrected by surgery. All men with diabetes over the age of 40 should have a prostate exam every year. If you have overflow incontinence, you may be able to manage the problem by reminding yourself to urinate on a schedule every day. If you continue to have trouble, you should seek help from a bladder specialist called a urologist.

Chapter Six: Complications—Macro

Will lowering the fat in my diet reduce my risk for heart disease?

Type of fat	Effect on your body	In summary...
Saturated fat: animal fats, lard	increases cholesterol increases heart disease	☹
Monounsaturated fat: olive oil, canola oil, nuts, avocado	lowers cholesterol no effect on HDL (good cholesterol)	☺
Polyunsaturated fat: corn oil, safflower oil	lowers cholesterol positive and negative effect on HDL	☺

▼
TIP:

In most cases, yes. You will especially lower your risk if you lower the saturated fats. Fats fall into one of three groups:

Saturated fats: Increase cholesterol in your blood and the risk of heart disease. They are usually solid at room temperature and are found in animal fats (meat, butter, lard, bacon, cheese), coconut, palm, and palm kernel oils, dairy fats, and hydrogenated vegetable fats (such as vegetable shortening and stick margarine).

Monounsaturated fats: Lower total cholesterol, do not affect HDL levels, and may reduce triglyceride levels. Food sources are olive oil, peanut oil, canola oil, olives, avocados, and nuts (except walnuts, which are polyunsaturated).

Polyunsaturated fats: Lower cholesterol levels but may also lower HDL levels. Food sources are vegetable oils such as corn, safflower, soybean, sunflower, and cottonseed.

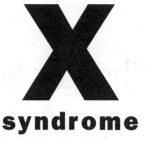

X
syndrome

*I*s my high blood pressure related
to my diabetes?

▼
TIP:

Probably. People with diabetes are more likely to have high
blood pressure. And people with the following symptoms
are more likely to develop diabetes or heart disease. The
combination of high blood pressure, high blood fat levels
(triglycerides), obesity (primarily in the abdominal region),
and insulin resistance is commonly called "Syndrome X." It is
not a specific disease but a group of related risk factors that
often exist together. The person with Syndrome X is at a
higher risk of developing diabetes and heart disease. Syndrome
X is very common and may affect up to 25% of all middle-
aged American males (and less commonly, females). So, to
answer your question, high blood pressure and diabetes are
related and often occur in the same individual. The important
health message is that a person with Syndrome X should
immediately seek medical advice to reduce his or her weight
and blood pressure. You should not wait until you develop diabetes or heart disease to change to a healthier lifestyle.

Chapter Seven:
MISCELLANEOUS

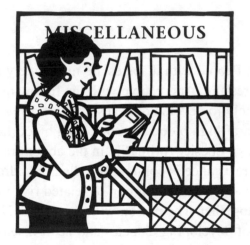

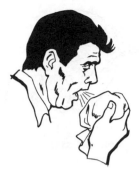

What can I take for a cough that is caused by my ACE inhibitor medication?

▼
TIP:

Many persons with diabetes have blood pressure problems. The Angiotensin Converting Enzyme (ACE) inhibitor blood pressure medications are ideal for this problem. One of their side benefits is to reduce pressure in the kidneys and to protect them from damage. Studies have shown that these medications actually reduce the rate of kidney damage caused by diabetes. Unfortunately, these drugs also affect the lungs, and about 20% of people treated with them develop an annoying cough. Although this cough is not dangerous, some patients have to stop taking their ACE inhibitor medication because they can't tolerate the cough. Losartan (Cozaar®), a new type of ACE inhibitor, has recently been approved by the Food and Drug Administration. This drug has many of the benefits of the ACE inhibitors on your blood pressure and kidneys, but it does not cause a cough. Ask your health-care team if this might be a good medication for you.

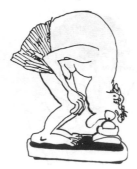

Why do I gain weight as I get older?

▼
TIP:

Unfortunately, most people do gain weight as they get older. There are several reasons. As you get older, your activity level changes to less strenuous exercise. For example, in the 20 to 30 year-old age group, many people jog, play tennis, work out at health clubs, etc. In later years, people change activities to include golf, bowling, and watching television. As your activities change, you burn fewer calories. If you're still eating the same amount of food that you always have, weight gain will follow. In addition, recent studies have suggested that older people are actually more efficient at storing food as fat. This means that for the same amount of food eaten, more exercise is needed to use it up. Thus, you should gradually decrease the amount of food that you eat as you get older in order to keep your body weight normal. In general, the leaner you are, the longer you will live.

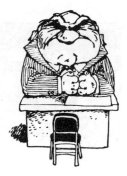

*C*an my diabetes cause constipation?

▼
TIP:

Y es. Constipation is the most common gastrointestinal dis-
order in people with diabetes, affecting about one in four
patients. Your chances of having constipation increase to 50%
if you have nerve problems due to diabetes. Most constipation
in people with diabetes is due to failure of the nerves which
control the muscles of the bowel or large intestine to work
properly. Other possible causes include blockage by a large
amount of hard, dry stool; low levels of thyroid hormone; or
an undiagnosed tumor. If you have frequent problems, you
should ask your health-care team for a complete evaluation of
your bowel, including thyroid hormone tests. This evaluation
may include a diagnostic test called a barium enema or a procedure where a stomach and intestinal specialist (gastroen-
terologist) inspects your bowel with a fiber-optic viewing
device (a colonoscope). If it turns out that your constipation is
due to diabetes alone, then you may get relief from the addition of fiber to your diet (psyllium colloid) or a gentle laxative,
such as docusate. You should not need even occasional enemas
if the above suggestions are followed.

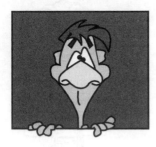

*S*hould *I be concerned about a blood pressure of 128/86?*

▼
TIP:

The most recent American Heart Association guidelines suggest that diastolic blood pressure (the bottom number) above 85 puts you at increased risk. Even mild elevations in blood pressure like yours increase the risk of complications such as retinopathy, nephropathy, and heart disease. You should discuss these readings with your health-care team. If your blood pressure readings are consistently high, you may need to start on blood pressure medication. Your doctor may ask you to check your blood pressure many times and in different settings to determine if your blood pressure is high all the time or goes up only at specific times. If you haven't tried exercise and diet to decrease your blood pressure, it's time to start a walking program and to decrease the sodium in your diet. The recommended amount of sodium is 2,400 mg/day or less. Start by taking away salt at the table. Read labels on foods to identify (and then reduce) the high sodium foods in your diet. Canned goods and prepared foods may be high in sodium. Drinking alcohol can also raise your blood pressure.

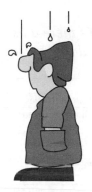

How do I handle the depression of having had diabetes for 25 years?

▼
TIP:

Depression is a common condition in people with chronic diseases like diabetes. Recognizing the symptoms of depression and making the diagnosis are keys to treating it A lack of energy, changes in eating habits, changes in sleep patterns (sleep disturbances which may lead to daytime drowsiness), and loss of interest in activities that you previously enjoyed are all symptoms that point to depression. You may lose interest in your diabetes management activities when you are depressed. It is important to talk to your health-care team about these feelings and changes in your life. Your physician may be able to recommend counselling or temporarily prescribe a medication which can help you enjoy life again.

*I*s there a list of tests and other things I am supposed to be doing to stay healthy?

Diabetes Checklist			
Care Activities	Frequency	Date	Date
Diabetes Control	Review BG log quarterly HbA$_{1c}$ goal _____		
Ophthalmology	Annual dilated exam Glaucoma, cataract check		
Renal	Proteinuria/microalbuminuria screen BUN/Creatinine annual		
Neuropathy/Feet	Feet and legs quarterly Podiatry referral		
Cardiovascular Exam	BP quarterly Lipids: annual screen fasting EKG baseline		
Hypoglycemia/ Hyperglycemia	Review management plan Glucagon on hand?		
Vaccinations	Flu: annual Pneumovax		
Diabetes Education	Initial & annual review		
Other:	Hospitalizations: Dates reason:		

▼

TIP:

Yes. The American Diabetes Association publishes "Standards of Medical Care For Patients with Diabetes Mellitus" to provide guidelines for health professionals to manage diabetes and prevent complications. We use a chart based on those standards to help our patients keep track of all that needs to be done. Some tests come every 3 months and some yearly. For instance, you should have your eyes checked by an ophthalmologist and your urine checked for microalbuminuria (small amounts of protein) yearly. With these two tests, your doctor can detect eye and kidney problems early and start treatment. You may want to keep track on your own flow sheet to be sure you get the tests done at the right time and to be able to share these results with your health-care team. Talk with them about which of these tests you need and when you should have each one done.

*W*hy *do I sleep all the time*
and yet never feel rested?

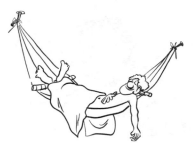

▼
TIP:

There are a number of reasons for someone to feel tired and want to sleep all the time. If your blood sugar is too high, it may make you very sleepy and lack energy. You may get very sleepy after eating a meal, a feeling which might be caused by an increase in your blood sugar. Your tiredness may be a side effect from your medications. Medicines associated with making you feel tired are some ulcer medications, antihistamines, blood pressure medications, treatment for stomach emptying problems (gastroparesis), and most antidepressants. Ask your pharmacist or physician if any of your medications may be causing your tiredness. You may have a thyroid problem that shows up as tiredness. Finally, you may be depressed and not realize it. Many people with depression sleep excessive numbers of hours and yet never feel rested. Other symptoms of depression include loss of appetite, disinterest in activities that you once enjoyed, and frequent crying spells. Talk to your health-care team about these symptoms. There are simple ways to identify depression, and good treatments available.

Why does a doctor have to sign my driver's license application?

▼

TIP:

This is so doctors can identify people who should not be driving for medical reasons. People with diabetes may endanger themselves and others if their eyesight is badly impaired due to diabetic eye disease. They may also suffer from frequent and severe low blood sugars which may interfere with their ability to operate an automobile. This risk is low, however, with only one out of every 10,000 automobile accidents being attributable to low blood sugar (a rate that is 1,000 times less than the risk of an alcohol-related accident). The best general approach to renewing your driver's license is to establish a relationship with your health-care team so that they know how well you manage your diabetes. In most cases, your physician will review your files and sign the form, agreeing that your license should be renewed. If there is a question about your eyesight, you may be sent to an eye doctor for evaluation. If your doctor feels that your blood sugar control is too erratic for you to operate an automobile safely, you may need to learn more about managing your diabetes responsibly. The potential loss of your driver's license may become the motivator you need to take charge of your diabetes!

*W*hy does it hurt when my
husband and I have sex?

▼
TIP:

Although men with diabetes more commonly have sexual problems, women may also experience sexual difficulties caused by the disease. These problems may include a decrease in sexual desire, vaginal dryness and pain with intercourse, or inability to achieve orgasm. Complaints such as these are not unique to people with diabetes but tend to occur more often in women with diabetes, especially those who are past menopause. Loss of sexual desire may be a symptom of depression. It frequently responds to medication or a few visits with a therapist. Some women have an increase in sexual desire after treatment with low dose testosterone (a hormone). Your pain during intercourse, however, most likely is caused by vaginal dryness and failure of your sex organs to adequately prepare for the sex act. If you are entering or past menopause, this problem may improve with estrogen replacement therapy or an estrogen cream which you apply intra-vaginally. The use of sexual lubricants may also greatly improve your enjoyment of sex. Talking about your concern with your health-care team may help you resume a fulfilling and mutually satisfying sex life with your husband.

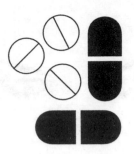

*I*s there any birth control method that
is preferred because I have diabetes?

▼
TIP:

You should use some kind of birth control if you are sexually active and don't want to get pregnant. Birth control
pills contain very low levels of estrogen (a hormone), and you
can use them. You may need more insulin, because the hormones in the birth control pills might make you a bit more
insulin resistant. A combination pill with norgestinate and a
synthetic estrogen is the best one for women with diabetes.
Foam, condoms, or a diaphragm work as long as they're used
every time. Condoms also provide the extra benefit of protection from sexually transmitted diseases, such as HIV. If you
want a birth control method that requires little effort, there
are hormone "implants" and injections. These provide birth
control over a longer period of time, but they do affect your
diabetes control. Another option for some women is the IUD
(intrauterine device), which is a small plastic device placed
inside the uterus that prevents implantation of fertilized eggs.
Because they can cause infections, they are not recommended
for women with diabetes.

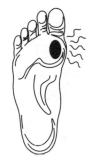

If my feet don't hurt, should I still check them every day?

▼
TIP:

Yes!! You should examine your feet at the end of each day to be certain that there are no sores, cuts, or areas where your shoe is rubbing against your foot. Because people with diabetes may lose pain sensation in their feet, they may develop ulcers and open sores and not notice them because they do not hurt. Without medical attention, sores may continue to be irritated and not heal properly. Although your health-care team should examine your feet at each visit, you need to be on the lookout for any small areas of redness or bleeding. Shoes that are comfortable and fit well are essential. Special shoes can be made for you if your feet are difficult to fit. Always wear socks or stockings to provide padding between your feet and your shoes. The longer a patient has diabetes, the more common foot problems are. Preventing foot sores is much easier than trying to heal them.

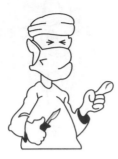

My doctor says that I should have my gallbladder removed, but isn't there a high risk of surgical complications due to my diabetes?

▼
TIP:

Patients with diabetes are at a higher risk of complications during and after a surgical procedure, but many such patients undergo successful surgery every day. Assuming that your surgery is necessary, then it is most important that your surgeon and your diabetes doctor work together before the surgery is performed to prevent problems. You should have a thorough medical checkup of your heart and kidneys, and you should make sure that your blood sugar control is good over the weeks prior to surgery. You should also be sure that you have had plenty of fluids to drink before reporting to the hospital. During the surgery, your doctors may control your blood sugar with intravenous insulin and glucose. Your diabetes doctor may even wish to be present during the surgery. After surgery, tight blood sugar control helps you reduce the risk of postoperative infections. By taking these precautions, you will have the best chances for a successful operation.

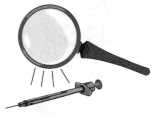

*H*ow accurately can I measure
*1/2-unit doses of insulin for my
2-year-old son who has diabetes?*

▼
TIP:

It is helpful to use low-dose (50 unit) or very low-dose (30 unit) syringes when measuring small amounts of insulin, since these syringes are narrower and have an expanded scale on the barrel. Syringe attachments which magnify and make it easier to read the scale are also available in many pharmacies. And, insulin manufacturers will provide diluting fluid if necessary for more accurate measurement.

Many children are extremely sensitive to insulin, and it is not unusual for doctors to prescribe 1/2-unit doses of Regular insulin for such patients. One recent study determined how accurately the parents (caretakers) of young children with diabetes were able to prepare very small doses of insulin. The results of this study suggest that people do not measure insulin very accurately in 1/2-unit doses. Interestingly, the study also found that people tend to overestimate the dose and deliver more insulin than they are supposed to. The good news is that each person tends to overestimate by the same amount nearly every time. So small children with diabetes may need to have only one caretaker who prepares their insulin injections to keep measurements consistent.

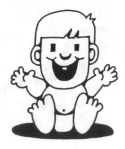

*W̶hat are the risks to my baby
  during my pregnancy?*

▼
TIP:

Pregnancy in diabetes carries risks for both you and your baby. Babies born of diabetic mothers have higher rates of birth defects and stillbirth. They can also be abnormally large, which complicates the delivery. You can avoid many of these problems by achieving near-normal blood sugar control before and during pregnancy. For example, infants born of diabetic mothers have about a 10% chance of being born with a birth defect, compared with only 2% of babies born to non-diabetic mothers. These birth defects typically involve the spinal cord, the kidneys, and the heart. This risk of birth defects can be greatly reduced, however, by achieving normal blood sugar control before pregnancy even occurs. In fact, blood sugar control is most important during the first 12 weeks of pregnancy because this is the time when all of the infant's major organs are formed. To be safe, you should plan on achieving a glycosylated hemoglobin level (HbA_{1c}) within 1% of normal before trying to get pregnant. If successful, you will give your baby the best chance for a healthy start in life, and you will also decrease the chances of delivering a very large baby. This will improve your chances of staying healthy, too.

If I am hospitalized, what should I expect regarding my diabetes care?

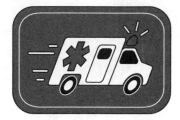

▼
TIP:

Your blood sugar control may worsen in the hospital due to varying meals and timing, inactivity, stress of being in the hospital, and changes in your insulin dose. The physician might not know your diabetes as well as you do. Stay involved in your diabetes care (assuming that you feel well enough). Measure your blood sugar yourself and keep a record by your bedside so you can discuss your sugars with your doctor. Your blood sugar should be measured at least four times a day. Your doctor should establish a target range for you, usually less than 200 mg/dl. Expect your insulin or oral diabetes medication at a reasonable time (at least 30 to 60 minutes before meals). If you feel that you are not getting enough food, ask for more and tell your doctor. If you are unable to eat, expect your diabetes to be controlled by insulin given in your vein. This will require frequent monitoring of your blood sugar to ensure that it does not go too low or too high. You should also expect the doctor to check your urine ketones more frequently in the hospital than you do at home, because fasting and stress can both lead to ketoacidosis. Taking an active role in your own diabetes care in the hospital will increase your chances of staying healthy.

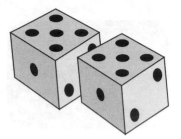

If I have "impaired glucose tolerance," what are my chances of getting diabetes later in life?

▼
TIP:

Consider impaired glucose tolerance to be a dangerous pre-diabetic condition. Reversing it with diet and exercise may prevent you from getting diabetes. Impaired glucose tolerance (IGT) is a gray area between having normal blood sugar and having diabetes. If you have IGT, your pre-breakfast blood sugar values are slightly elevated, usually above 110 mg/dl. This level is not high enough to qualify for a diagnosis of diabetes, which is above 140 mg/dl. Although you don't have diabetes, 5% of people with IGT do develop diabetes every year. This means that if you have had IGT for five years, your chances for getting diabetes increase to about 25%. People with IGT are overweight, don't get much exercise, and usually have relatives who have type II diabetes. Most doctors believe that if people with IGT improve their health by losing weight and getting more exercise, their chance for developing diabetes will be much lower. Also, eating a low-fat and high-fiber diet may help. You should get your blood sugar level checked at least once a year and if it is high, go to work on getting it into the normal range and keeping it there.

Chapter Eight:
RESOURCES

Manufacturers listed in this section can provide tips for proper use of their products.

To request more information about other books published by the American Diabetes Association, write to:

American Diabetes Association
Order Fulfillment Department
P.O. Box 930850
Atlanta, GA 31193-0850

or call (800) ADA-ORDER

American Association of Diabetes Educators . . . . . .(800) 338-3633
444 N. Michigan Ave.   (312) 644-2233
Suite 1240
Chicago, IL 60611-3901

American Diabetes Association . . . .(800) 806-7801
Patient Information   (800) 342-2383
1660 Duke St.   (703) 549-1500
Alexandria, VA 22314

American Dietetic Association . . . .(800) 366-1655
216 West Jackson Blvd.
Suite 800
Chicago, IL 60606-6995

Bayer Corporation . . . .(800) 348-8100
511 Benedict Ave.
Tarrytown, NY 10591

Becton Dickinson Consumer Products . . . .(800) 237-4554
One Becton Dr.
Building #2
Franklin Lakes, NJ 07417-1883

Boehringer Mannheim Corporation . . . .(800) 858-8072
9115 Hague Rd.
P.O. Box 50100
Indianapolis, IN 46250-0100

Chronimed, Inc. . . . .(800) 444-5951
Ridgedale Office Center, Suite 250   (612) 541-0239
13911 Ridgedale Dr.
Minneapolis, MN 55305

Cascade Medical . . . .(612) 941-7345
10180 Viking Drive   (800) 525-6718
Eden Prairie, MN 55344

Eli Lilly and Company . . . .(800) 545-5979
Lilly Corporate Center   (317) 276-2000
Indianapolis, IN 46285

Home Diagnostics, Inc. . . . .(800) 342-7226
2300 NW 55th Ct.   (305) 677-9201
Ft. Lauderdale, FL 33309

International Diabetic Athletes Association . . . .(602) 230-8155
6829 North 12th St., Ste. 205
Phoenix, AZ 85014

Lifescan, Inc. . . . .(800) 227-8862
1000 Gilbraltar Dr.   (408) 263-9789
Milpitas, CA 95035-6312

MediSense, Inc. . . . .(800) 527-3339
266 Second Ave.
Waltham, MA 02154

Minimed Technologies . . . .(800) 933-3322
12744 San Fernando Rd.
Sylmar, CA 91342

National Diabetes Information Clearinghouse . . . . .(301) 468-2162
Box NDIC
9000 Rockville Pk.
Bethesda, MD 20892

Novo Nordisk Pharmaceuticals, Inc. . . . .(800) 727-6500
100 Overlook Center   (609) 987-5800
Suite 200
Princeton, NJ 08540

Polymer Technology International . . . .(800) 877-4449
1871 NW Gilman Blvd.
Issaquah, WA 98027

INDEX

Bones, infections in, 22

C

Camps, 30
Capsaicin, 74
Cataracts, 68
Causes of diabetes, 3, 16, 19, 108
Certified Diabetes Educator (CDE), 11
Children
  blood glucose control and, 29
  coping with diabetes, 29–30, 41
  diabetes summer camps for, 30
  insulin dosage for, 105
Chocolate
  craving for, 57
  gustatory sweating and, 78
Cholesterol
  fat intake and, 90
  heart disease and, 87
Cholestyramine, 24
Chromium supplements, 48
Cigarette smoking, 81
COBRA benefits, 18
Cold medicines, 31
Collip, James, 10
Complications. *See also* individual complications
  macro, 80–91
  micro, 67–78
  prevention of, 44, 70
Condoms, 102
Conjunctivitis, viral, 72
Constipation, 95
Contagiousness, of diabetes, 3
Contraceptives, 38, 102
Coping with diabetes. *See also* Depression
  children and, 29–30, 41
Cortisol, 40
Cough medicines, 31
Coughs, from ACE inhibitor medication, 93
Coworkers, diabetes disclosure and, 2
Cow's milk, as trigger for diabetes, 19
Cozaar, 93
Cures, for diabetes, 4, 12, 39
Cysteine, 53

101 Tips for Staying Healthy with Diabetes (& Avoiding Complications)

D

Deaths
  diabetes-related, 13
  from heart disease, 84
Decongestants, 31
Depression, 32
  children and, 41
  sex drive and, 83, 101
  symptoms of, 97, 99
Diabetes centers, 11
Diabetes mellitus, origin of term, 14
Diabetic gastroparesis, 71
Diabetic kidney disease. *See also* Kidneys
  pregnancy and, 69, 73
Diarrhea, 24
Diet. *See also* Supplements, dietary
  chocolate, 57
  fats, 90
  fiber, 49
  food guide pyramid, 60
  food labels, 59
  fructose, 50
  health foods, 49–55
  and IGT, reversing, 108
  meal plans. *See* Meal planning
  protein, 76
  sodium intake, lowering, 58
  weight reduction programs, 61
Dipyridamole stress test, 84
Disclosure, of diabetes, 2
Dizziness, 82
Doctor visits
  checklist for, 98
  frequency of, 7, 68, 89, 98
  for heart disease screening, 84
  preparation for, 6
Docusate, 95
Driving
  blood glucose testing before, 43
  commercial vehicles, insulin use and, 25
  license renewal, 100

E

Erections, maintaining, 83

Erythromycin, 24
Estrogen, 101
Exercise
  arthritis and, 33
  athletic shoes, 80
  benefits, 33
  blood glucose testing before, 43
  to decrease blood pressure, 96
  and IGT, reversing, 108
  laser therapy and, 77
  stopping medication and, 45
Eye problems, 68
  assessments, 7
  blindness, 13, 68, 72
  glaucoma, 72
  infections, 72
  pregnancy and, 69
  temporary loss of vision, 82

F
Fainting spells, 82
Family members, reading this book, 8
Fat, dietary, 90
Fatigue, 36, 97, 99
Fiber, dietary, 49, 95
  diabetic gastroparesis and, 71
Finger joints, stiffness in, 74
Fingernails, fungal infections of, 20
Finger sticks, reducing pain of, 35
Floaters, 68
Florinef, 82
Folate, 53
Folic acid, 53
Food and Drug Administration, 15, 21, 52, 59
Food guide pyramid, 60
Food labeling, 59
Foot care, 22, 85–86
  athlete's foot, 20
  daily examination, 103
  painful neuropathy, 74
  shoes, 80, 103
Frank, Johann Peter, 14
Fructose, 50
Fungal infections, 20, 23

G

Ginseng, 51–52
Glaucoma, 72
Glipizide, 46
Glucophage, 21
Glucose control. *See* Blood glucose levels
Glucose sensors, 4
Glucose testing. *See* Blood glucose testing
Glyburide, 46
Glycosylated hemoglobin (HbA$_{1c}$), 67
  level for pregnancy, 106
Gustatory sweating, 78

H

Hands, stiffness in, 75
Health-care team, 11. *See also* Doctor visits
Health foods, 49–55
Health insurance
  pancreas transplants and, 39
  pre-existing condition exclusion, 18
Health management. *See also* Doctor visits
  coworkers and, 2
  test guidelines, 98
Heart disease
  cholesterol and, 87
  fat intake and, 90
  homocysteine and, 53
  hot tubs and, 88
  risk of, 81, 91
  saunas and, 88
  Syndrome X, 91
  testing for, 84
  waist/hip ratio and, 65
Hemoglobin, glycosylated, 67, 106
Hepatitis, 35
Herbal remedies, 52
Heredity, as cause of diabetes, 3, 16
High blood glucose. *See also* Blood glucose levels
  damage from, 44
Historical background, diabetes, 10, 14
Homocysteine, 53
Hospitalization
  blood glucose control and, 107
  surgery, 104

Hot tubs, 88

I
Impaired glucose tolerance (IGT), 108
Incontinence, 89
Infections
  eye, 72
  foot, 22, 86
  from IUDs, 102
  postoperative, 104
  skin, 23
Infectiousness, of diabetes, 3
Insoluble fiber, 49
Insulin
  allergic reaction to, 42
  birth control pills and, 102
  blood glucose testing and, 43
  discovery of, 10
  driving commercial vehicles and, 25
  low dosages for children, 105
  weight gain and, 46
Insulin-dependent diabetes. *See* Type I diabetes
Insulin pumps, 4, 37
Internet, diabetes information on, 27
IUD (intrauterine device), 102

J
Juvenile Diabetes Foundation International, 12

K
Kaopectate, 24
Ketoacidosis, 26, 62, 107
Ketones, 26, 62, 107
Kidneys
  assessments of, 7
  blood pressure medication and, 93
  failure of, 13
  problems during pregnancy, 69, 73
  protein and, 76
  transplants of, 39

L
Langerhans, Paul, 10
Laser therapy, 68

exercise following, 77
Leg cramps, 74
Lomotil, 24
Loperamide, 24
Losartan, 93
Low blood glucose, 36. *See also* Blood glucose levels

M
Macular edema, 68
Magnesium supplements, 54
Meal planning. *See also* Diet
  adherence to, 63
  frequency of meals, 64
Medical costs, 18
  insulin pumps, 37
  pancreas transplants, 39
Medical visits. *See* Doctor visits
Medications *See also* individual medications
  for colds, 31
  contraceptives, 38
  for depression, 32
  for high blood pressure, 93
  new. *See* New products
  sexual problems and, 83
  stopping, 45
  tiredness and, 99
  weight gain and, 46
Melatonin, 55
Metamucil, 49
Metformin, 21
Meyer, Jean de, 10
Mineral supplements. *See* Supplements, dietary
Minkowski, Oskar, 10
Monounsaturated fats, 90

N
Nerve problems
  bladder function, 89
  constipation, 95
  gustatory sweating, 78
  painful neuropathy, 74
  postural dizziness, 82
New products, 15
  blood glucose levels and, 45

for blood pressure problems, 93
for complication prevention, 67
for Type II diabetes, 21
Nicotine patches, 81
Non insulin-dependent diabetes. *See* Type II diabetes
Nutrition. *See* Diet

O
Obesity, 91. *See also* Weight control

P
Painful neuropathy, 74
Pancreas, 4, 10, 16
  transplants, 39
Podiatrists (DPMs), 85–86
Polyunsaturated fats, 90
Postural dizziness, 82
Prayer sign, 75
Precose, 21
Prednisone, 40
Pregnancy
  blood glucose control and, 106
  diabetes during, 9
  high blood pressure and, 69
  kidney disease and, 73
  risks, 69
Prevention
  of complications, 44, 70
  of diabetes, 16, 108
Products, new. *See* New products
Prostate exams, 89
Protein, 76
Pseudophilin, 49
Psychological problems. *See* Depression
Psyllium, 24, 95
Puberty, 30

R
Retinopathy, 68, 77
Rollo, John, 14

S
Saturated fats, 90
Saunas, 88

Triglyceride levels, 90, 91
Type I diabetes
  causes of, 3, 16, 19
  ketoacidosis, 62
  occurrence, 17
  prevention of, 16
Type II diabetes
  causes of, 3, 16
  dietary fiber and, 49
  ginseng and, 51–52
  new therapies for, 20
  occurrence, 17
  prevention of, 16, 108
  stopping medication, 45

U
Urine leakage, 89
Urine testing, 26

V
Vaginal dryness, 101
Vanadium, 52
Viral conjunctivitis, 72
Vision. *See* Eye problems
Vitamin supplements. *See* Supplements, dietary

W
Waist/hip ratio, 65
Weight control, 46
  age and, 94
  diet/weight reduction programs, 61
  and IGT, reversing, 108
  obesity, 91
  Syndrome X, 90
  waist/hip ratio, 65
Weight Watchers, 61
White classification, 69
Wine, 34
World Wide Web, diabetes information on, 27

Y
Yawning, 36
Yeast infections, 23
Yohimbine, 83